AF352385

# Intravenous Immunoglobulin in Dermatology

*Edited by*

STEPHEN JOLLES MSc PhD MRCP MRCPath

LRF FELLOW & HONORARY CONSULTANT IN IMMUNOLOGY
& ALLERGY
NATIONAL INSTITUTE OF MEDICAL RESEARCH
AND ROYAL FREE HOSPITAL
LONDON
UK

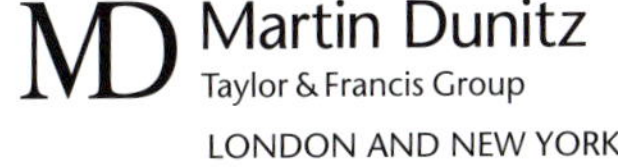


LONDON AND NEW YORK

First published in the United Kingdom in 2003 by
Martin Dunitz, an imprint of the Taylor & Francis Group, 11 New Fetter Lane,
London EC4P 4EE

Tel.:      +44 (0) 20 7583 9855
Fax.:      +44 (0) 20 7842 2298
E-mail:    info@dunitz.co.uk
Website:   http://www.dunitz.co.uk



A CIP record for this book is available from the British Library.

ISBN 1 84184 136 6

Distributed in the USA by
Fulfilment Center
Taylor & Francis
10650 Tobben Drive
Independence, KY 41051, USA
Toll Free Tel.: +1 800 634 7064
E-mail: taylorandfrancis@thomsonlearning.com

Distributed in Canada by
Taylor & Francis
74 Rolark Drive
Scarborough, Ontario M1R 4G2, Canada
Toll Free Tel.: +1 877 226 2237
E-mail: tal_fran@istar.ca

Distributed in the rest of the world by
Thomson Publishing Services
Cheriton House
North Way
Andover, Hampshire SP10 5BE, UK
Tel.: +44 (0)1264 332424
E-mail: salesorder.tandf@thomsonpublishingservices.co.uk

Composition by Wearset Ltd, Boldon, Tyne and Wear

Printed and bound in Italy by Printer Trento

# Contents


**Contributors**    *vii*

**Preface**    *ix*

**1**    **Intravenous immunoglobulins – mechanisms of action**    *1*
Hans-Peter Hartung and Bernd C Kieseier

**2**    **The role of high-dose intravenous immunoglobulin in dermatomyositis**    *21*
Marinos C Dalakas

**3**    **Chronic urticaria**    *33*
Brigid F O'Donnell

**4**    **Atopic dermatitis – role of hdIVIg**    *53*
Samantha Eisman and Malcolm HA Rustin

**5**    **Kawasaki disease**    *63*
Andrew J Cant and Laura Jones

**6**    **Toxic epidermal necrolysis**    *79*
Nicholas M Craven

**7 Intravenous immunoglobulin in the treatment of scleromyxoedema, scleroderma, pyoderma gangrenosum and pretibial myxoedema**     **93**
*Stephen Jolles*

**8 IVIg therapy in autoimmune mucocutaneous blistering diseases**     **107**
*A Razzaque Ahmed and Naveed Sami*

**9 Safety and tolerability of intravenous immunoglobulins**     **129**
*Turf D Martin*

**Index**     **145**

# Contributors

**A Razzaque Ahmed** MD
Department of Oral Medicine
Harvard School of Dental Medicine
Boston, MA
USA

**Andrew J Cant**
Paediatric Immunology & Infectious Diseases Unit
Newcastle General Hospital
Westgate Road
Newcastle upon Tyne
UK

**Nicholas M Craven**
Honorary Consultant Dermatologist
Dermatology Centre
Hope Hospital
Salford
Manchester
UK

**Marinos C Dalakas** MD
National Institutes of Neurological Disorders
and Stroke
National Institutes of Health
Bethesda, MD
USA

**Samantha Eisman** MBChB MRCP
Specialist Registrar in Dermatology
Royal Free Hospital
London
UK

**Hans-Peter Hartung** MD
Department of Neurology
Heinrich-Heine-University
Düsseldorf
Germany

**Laura Jones**
Clinical Research Fellow
Child Health
Sir James Spence Institute
Royal Victoria Infirmary,
Newcastle upon Tyne
UK

**Stephen Jolles** PhD MRCP MRCPath
LRF Fellow & Honorary Consultant in
Immunology & Allergy
National Institute of Medical Research and
Royal Free Hospital
London
UK

**Bernd C Kieseier** MD
Department of Neurology
Heinrich-Heine-University
Düsseldorf
Germany

**Turf D Martin**
Genesis Medical Marketing Consultants, LLC
Sedalia, Missouri
USA

**Brigid F O'Donnell** MD MRCPI DCH
Consultant Dermatologist
The Children's University Hospital
Temple Street, Dublin
Ireland

**Malcolm HA Rustin** MBChB FRCP
Consultant Dermatologist
Royal Free Hospital
London
UK

**Naveed Sami** MD
Department of Oral Medicine
Harvard School of Dental Medicine
Boston, MA
USA

# Preface

The major clinical specialties using intravenous immunoglobulin (IVIg) have been immunology, neurology and haematology. More recently, however, there has been an increase in the dermatological use of high dose IVIg (hdIVIg). This book is broadly based on a symposium held at the Dermatology 2000 meeting in Vienna, Austria and aims to provide a critical summary of the current data concerning the use of hdIVIg in the major dermatological conditions to which it has been applied.

HdIVIg is already an established treatment in some of these conditions such as Kawasaki disease and therapy resistant dermatomyositis, however the data in many others is derived from small studies and case reports. There are very few double-blind randomized studies of the use of hdIVIg in dermatological disorders and it is becoming clear that a number of the conditions described in this book have accrued sufficient evidence of benefit in smaller studies to warrant similarly designed studies. These studies will need to address a number of questions not only of efficacy but also which other agents should be chosen when hdIVIg is used adjunctively, what is the mechanism of action and how long should it be continued. Studies using IVIg in the treatment of inflammatory or autoimmune disease have led to a better understanding of the pathogenic mechanisms underlying these disorders and hence new potential treatment modalities. The future may see genetically engineered components of IVIg such as Fc or monoclonal antibodies used for specific indications. It is hoped that readers find the book helpful in distilling the current evidence for the use of hdIVIg in dermatological conditions as well as understanding its mechanism(s) of action in these diseases.

**Stephen Jolles**

# Intravenous immunoglobulins – mechanisms of action

## 1

**Hans-Peter Hartung and Bernd C Kieseier**

ADCC: antibody-dependent cellular cytotoxicity; IFN: interferon; LFA: lymphocyte function-associated antigen; MAC: membrane attack complex; MHC: major histocompatibility complex

Intravenous immunoglobulins (IVIg) were initially used as a replacement therapy in patients with hypogammaglobulinaemia. Fortuitously, in 1981 Imbach and colleagues[1] discovered that these preparations exhibited beneficial therapeutic effects in idiopathic thrombocytopenic purpura. Since this observation, IVIg has been tested at least experimentally in numerous disorders of presumed autoimmune genesis. Although the complete spectrum of mechanisms of action of IVIg is not yet completely understood, experimental and clinical studies have elucidated a number of mechanisms by which IVIg may modify disease. The following chapter aims to provide insight into the present status of knowledge on mechanisms of action of IVIg, based on immunological concepts relevant in the pathogenesis of immune-mediated disorders.

# Immunoglobulins in the immune system

The immune system is an organization of cells and molecules with specialized tasks in defending the organism from external agents, usually infectious but also toxic. Moreover, the immune system plays a pivotal role in maintaining antigenic homeostasis in the body.

Based on the formation of immunological memory, the immune system has traditionally been divided into *innate* and *adaptive* systems, each of which contains different cellular and molecular components and thus performs different functions. The main distinction between these two systems lies in the mechanisms and receptors used for immune recognition.[2,3]

The *adaptive* immune system is based on two classes of highly specialized cells, T and B lymphocytes. Each of these cells expresses a single kind of structurally unique receptor, resulting in a broad and extremely diverse repertoire of antigen recognition.

Both, B and T lymphocytes are derived from primordial stem cells in primary lymphoid tissues such as the bone marrow and the fetal liver. Their development is guided by interactions with stromal cells, such as fibroblasts, and cytokines, including various colony-stimulating factors. However, the early phase of lymphocyte development is not dependent on the presence of antigen, but

once these cells express a mature antigen receptor, their further differentiation and survival becomes antigen-dependent.

## B lymphocytes

The development of B lymphocytes is characterized by successive steps in the rearrangement and expression of immunoglobulin genes, as well as by changes in the expression of cell surface and intracellular molecules. In the bone marrow B cell development proceeds in the absence of an antigen until a complete IgM molecule is expressed on the surface of the cell, which is defined as an *immature B cell*. This cell population is subject to selection for self-tolerance and ability to survive in the periphery, a complex regulatory mechanism still not fully elucidated. After this selection immature B cells enter the periphery and access lymphoid follicles. The majority of these cells emerging from the bone marrow survive for less than a week, probably because of the competition for follicular access. The surviving cells form part of the long-lived pool of *mature peripheral B cells*. These lymphocytes, co-expressing IgM and IgD, recirculate through the lymphoid organs, until they encounter their specific antigen. Once the immunoglobulin receptor on the B cell surface interacts with a specific antigen, the B cell will be activated. This process requires a series of additional stimulatory signals besides the direct contact between antigen and B cell receptor. After antigen recognition the B cell is activated to divide. Selected B cells will differentiate into *plasma cells*, which secrete large amounts of immunoglobulin, or into long-lived *memory cells*, which contribute to lasting protective immunity.

Besides synthesizing specific antibodies B lymphocytes are capable of binding, internalizing, and digesting antigen, and can re-express the digested protein fragments on their cell surface in the context of major histocompatibility complex (MHC) proteins. As such, B cells can act as specific antigen-presenting cells as well.

## B cell receptor and soluble antibodies

The unique feature of B lymphocytes is their ability to express and secrete immunoglobulins or antibodies. Antibodies consist of two identical heavy chains and two identical light chains that are held together by disulphide bonds.[4] The N terminal of each chain possesses a variable domain that binds antigen through three hypervariable complementarity-determining regions. The C terminal domains of the heavy and the light chains form the constant regions, which define the class and subclass of the antibody and govern whether the light chain is of the κ or the λ type (Fig. 1.1). Five different classes of antibody (IgD, IgM, IgG, IgA and IgE),

four subclasses of IgG and two subclasses of IgA are known, each of which exhibits different functional properties (Table 1.1). Each type of antibody can be produced as a soluble circulating molecule or as a stationary molecule, the latter anchored through a transmembrane domain on the B-cell surface, where it acts as the *B-cell receptor.*

Most resting B lymphocytes express IgD and IgM molecules on their surface. The antigen response starts with binding of the antigen to IgM-expressing B cells, resulting in the production of antibodies of the same specificity. After antigen contact class switching will occur and most B cells will produce IgG immunoglobulins. During a secondary response to the same antigen a relative increase in IgG is observed. Depending on their environment, some B cells will synthesize IgA (preferentially in the gut) or IgE (especially in the lung and the skin). The determinants of class switching are not completely understood.

Antibody genes continually change as B cells encounter antigen and proliferate. Certain portions of the hypervariable regions are active sites of mutation, resulting in an ongoing refinement of the antibody response. Besides the increase in number of antibodies secreted, the affinity of individual antibodies against the stimulating antigen increases over time, as B cells expressing higher-affinity receptors on their surface are selectively activated. This process increases both the

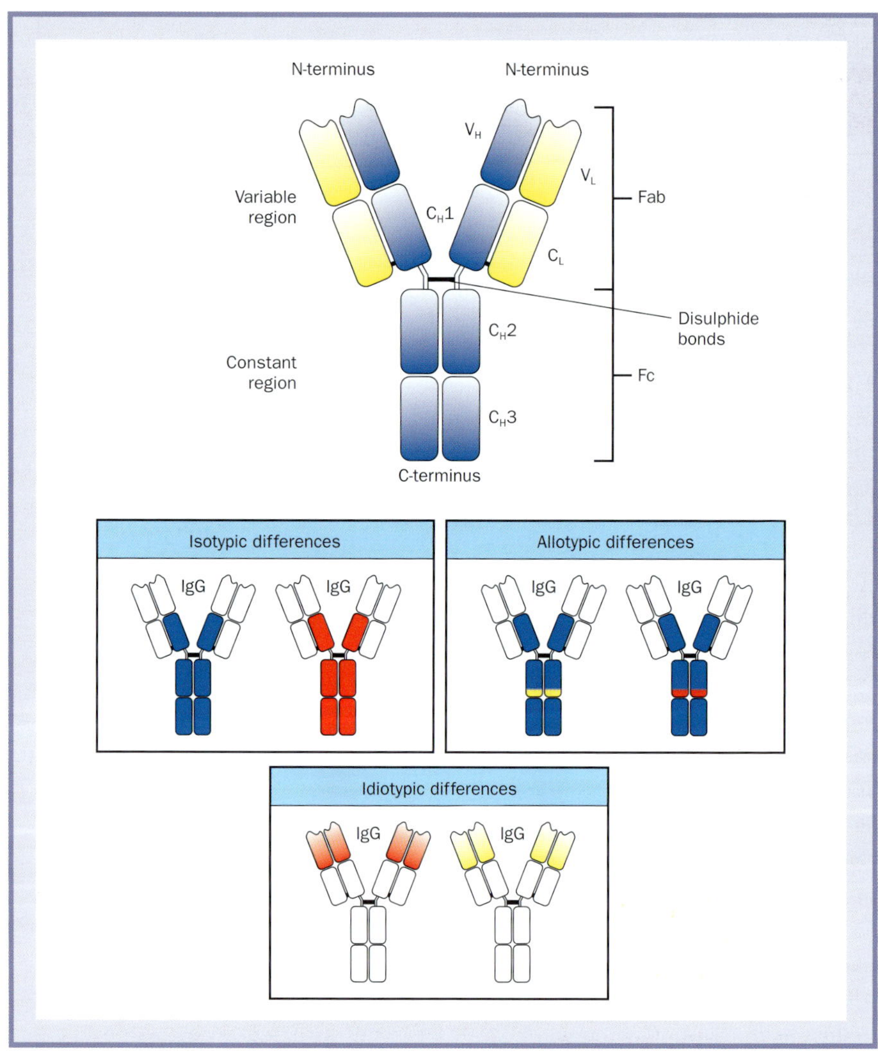


**Fig. 1.1**
*Basic structure of the IgG molecule (top panel) and its partial differentiation. Immunoglobulin isotypes are responsible for the biological effector functions of antibody molecules. Allotypes reflect the existence of two or more variants of a given gene encoding for immunoglobulins. The unique tertiary structure of the antigen-binding site of an antigen-specific receptor is referred to as the idiotype.*

**Table 1.1**
*Human immunoglobulin isotypes*

| | IgG1 | IgG2 | IgG3 | IgG4 | IgM | IgA1 | IgA2 | IgD | IgE |
|---|---|---|---|---|---|---|---|---|---|
| **Structure** | | | | | | | | | |
| Heavy chain | $\gamma1$ | $\gamma2$ | $\gamma3$ | $\gamma4$ | $\mu$ | $\alpha1$ | $\alpha2$ | $\delta$ | $\varepsilon$ |
| Molecular weight (kDa) | 146 | 146 | 165 | 146 | 970 | 160 | 160 | 184 | 188 |
| Half-life in serum (days) | 21 | 20 | 7 | 21 | 10 | 6 | 6 | 3 | 2 |
| | | | | | | | | | |
| **Function** | | | | | | | | | |
| Activation of classic complement pathway | ++ | + | +++ | – | +++ | – | – | – | – |
| Activation of alternative complement pathway | – | – | – | – | – | + | – | – | – |
| Binding to macrophages/ phagocytes | + | – | + | – | – | + | + | – | + |
| Binding to mast cells/basophils | – | – | – | – | – | – | – | – | +++ |

efficiency and the specificity of the immune response.

The functions of immunoglobulins are manifold but essentially serve to neutralize foreign antigens. In various immune-mediated disorders the entire functional spectrum of humoral immunity can be observed: antibody binding to cellular surfaces results in complement activation and, consequently, tissue destruction. The recognition of antibody-coated peptides by accessory effector cells triggers the activation of macrophages, resulting in the release of inflammatory mediators in the surrounding tissue and so perpetuating local inflammation. Moreover, antibodies binding to target antigens can, via Fc receptors, activate a toxic programme called antibody-dependent cellular cytotoxicity (ADCC), directing an antigen-specific attack by an effector cell through the cellular release of cytoplasmic granules containing granzymes or perforins.[5]

# Intravenous immunoglobulins – preparations

Commercially available IVIg preparations are derived from a human plasma pool of 2000–5000 healthy donors.[6] Such a large donor pool ensures that the diversity of immunoglobulins in the preparation far exceeds the repertoire of a single human being: this is sometimes referred to as a 'species repertoire'. Such diversity may be important for the therapeutic effect. Differences in manufacture may influence the therapeutic effect, side effects and safety of the IVIg preparation.[7–9] Preparations for intravenous application contain IgG almost exclusively, with only traces of other immunoglobulins or aggregates.[10] The distribution of the four IgG subclasses generally equates to that in normal serum, but differences between various commercial preparations are described.[11–13] IVIg has been shown to contain 40% dimers and 60% monomers.

Moreover, traces of other immunologically active molecules, such as soluble HLA molecules,[14] soluble CD4 and CD8[15] and IgA, have been reported to be present in IVIg.[10] Although the relevance of these other potentially immunologically active molecules needs to be critically discussed, the amounts of these substances vary between manufacturers and it remains difficult to assess to what extent this remains important for the therapeutic effect.[16] At present the various IVIg preparations are generally considered therapeutically equivalent and interchangeable.[17]

# Intravenous immunoglobulins – mechanisms of action

Disturbances in the finely tuned interactions between helper and suppressor T lymphocytes, B lymphocytes, immunoglobulin producing plasma cells, macrophages, dendritic cells and other effector cells are thought to play a key role in the pathogenesis of immune-mediated disorders (Table 1.2). The mechanisms of anti-inflammatory effects of IVIg are manifold.[18]

## *Suppression of antibody production*

One of the mechanisms first suggested to mediate the beneficial effects of IVIg was the downregulation of antibody production, including autoantibodies, by B lymphocytes. IgG binds via its Fc fragment to corresponding cellular surface receptors. Cross-linking of neighbouring Fc receptors by IgG has been demonstrated to effectively induce negative signals to B cells, resulting in a reduction of immunoglobulin synthesis.[19–20] Recent data suggest that both Fc and Fab portions contribute to the inhibition of immunoglobulin production, specifically IgE.[21]

A specific subset of B cells (B1 cells) identifiable by the surface antigen CD5 has been shown to produce autoantibodies with low affinity. These antibodies form part of the natural repertoire available to any individual. It has been demonstrated that IVIg preparations contain antibodies to CD5, and may thereby potentially downregulate the production of pathogenic autoantibodies (Fig. 1.2).[22,23] In atopic dermatitis IVIg therapy was shown to increase serum levels of soluble

**Table 1.2**
*Immunomodulatory mechanisms of IVIg*

| Component of the immune system | Function modulated/mechanism postulated | Refs |
| --- | --- | --- |
| *Fc receptor* | *Inhibition of Fc receptor-mediated phagocytosis*<br>*Accelerated elimination of autoantibodies via Fc receptor neonate (FcRn)*<br>*Blockade of antibody-dependent macrophage-mediated cellular cytotoxicity cross–linkage*<br>*FcγRIIB required to exhibit immunomodulation* | *1, 18, 25, 33–35* |
| *Complement* | *Binding of C1, C3b, and C4b*<br>*Inactivation of complement–IgG complexes*<br>*Saturation of CR1 and CR3 receptors on activated macrophages* | *31–32* |
| *Anti-idiotypic antibodies* | *Neutralization of autoantibodies* | *26–30* |
| *Cytokines* | *Modulation of cytokine production (favouring Th1 over Th2)*<br>*Trace amounts of IFN-γ and TGF-β*<br>*Antibodies against various cytokines*<br>*Protective effect against TNF-α-mediated damage* | *39–43* |
| *T cells* | *Antibodies against T-cell receptor, HLA class I*<br>*Antibodies against LFA-1 accessory molecule*<br>*Antibodies against activating superantigens*<br>*Soluble CD4 and HLA I/II molecules*<br>*Enhanced suppressor T-cell function*<br>*Alter cell cycling and apoptosis* | *38, 46–52* |
| *B cells* | *Anti-idiotypic antibodies*<br>*Anti-CD5 antibodies: inactivation of autoantibody-producing CD20⁺(B1) B-cell subset*<br>*Inhibition of antibody production* | *19–23, 26-30* |
| *Cell adhesion* | *Inhibits migration of immunocompetent cells into target tissue* | *46* |
| *Glucocorticoid receptor* | *Increases receptor sensitivity* | *56* |

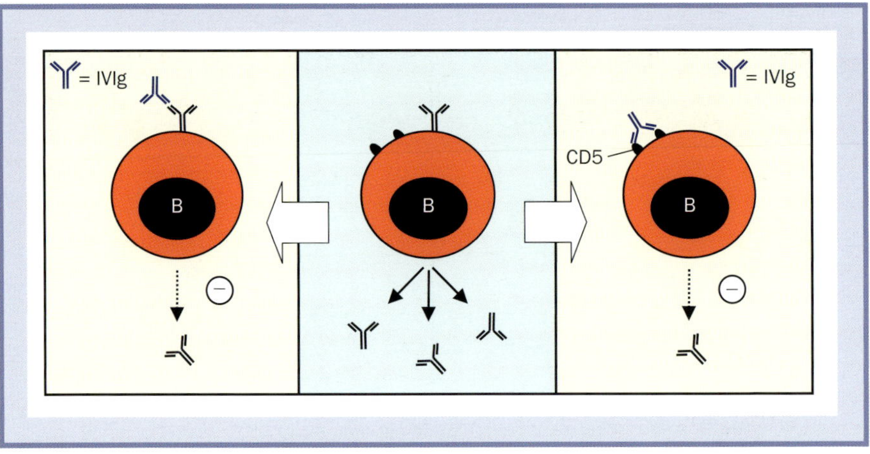


**Fig. 1.2**
*Accelerated metabolism and downregulation of the synthesis of autoantibodies. IVIg have been proposed to induce the catabolism of endogenous IgG (left panel). A specific subset of B cells, identified by the expression of the surface antigen CD5, releases antibodies of low affinity but high avidity. IVIg preparations contain antibodies to CD5 and may thereby potentially downregulate the production of pathogenic autoantibodies (right panel).*

CD5, but the functional implication of this observation remains elusive at present.[24]

## Acceleration of antibody catabolism

It has been observed that the application of IVIg results in a reduced half-life of circulating immunoglobulin. A potential mechanism based on an accelerated catabolism of endogenous IgG, including pathogenic IgG, has been proposed. IgG binding to a protective receptor on endocytotic vesicles, termed FcRn, prevents lysosomal degradation of IgG. Saturation of this receptor by IVIg may result in the escape of endogenous IgG from these protective mechanisms, resulting in accelerated antibody catabolism.[25]

## Neutralization of autoantibodies

As indicated above, IVIg preparations represent a diverse repertoire of immunoglobulins. They contain 'anti-idiotypic' antibodies that can bind and neutralize pathogenic antibodies, maintaining the immune homeostasis in an idiotype–anti-idiotype network (Fig. 1.3).[22, 26–29] Clinically, this effect was observed by Kazatchkine and

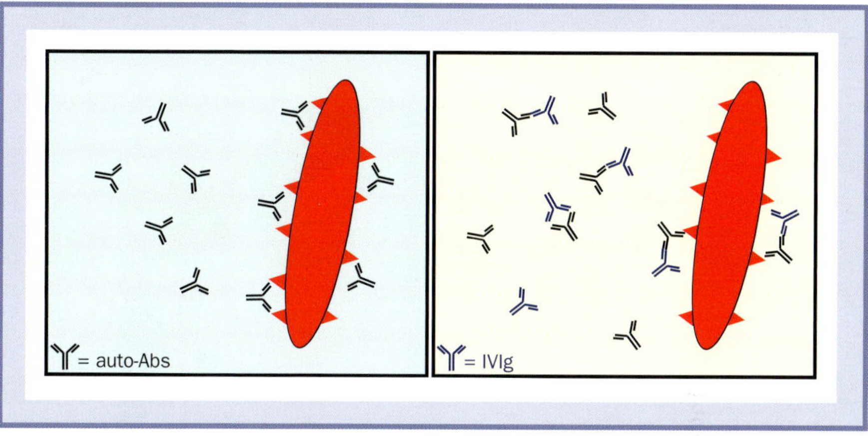



**Fig. 1.3**
*IVIg preparations contain anti-idiotypic antibodies that can bind and neutralize pathogenic antibodies.*

co-workers when they treated patients with autoantibodies to factor VIII with intravenous γ-globulins. After IVIg a marked reduction or disappearance of these antibodies was found. Sultan et al. demonstrated that the γ-globulin preparations contained anti-idiotypic antibodies to the anti-factor VIII antibodies.[30]

## Neutralization of complement-mediated effects

Activation of the complement system is one mechanism through which antibodies mediate deleterious tissue damage. During the process of complement activation various proinflammatory peptides, such as C3a and C5a, phagocytosis-promoting factors such as

C3b, as well as the assembly of the membrane attack complex (MAC) made up of the terminal complement components C5b-9, are released. MAC can permeabilize membranes, precipitating an influx of calcium that in turn can activate membrane-integral proteases (Fig. 1.4).

In guinea pigs the so-called Forssman antigen is widely distributed on endothelial cells. The intravenous application of antibodies to Forssman antigen results in the development of irreversible shock and death. May and Frank[31] demonstrated that guinea pigs genetically deficient in the fourth component of complement (C4) did not sustain shock upon intravenous administration of Forssman antibody but that this reaction could be restored in animals

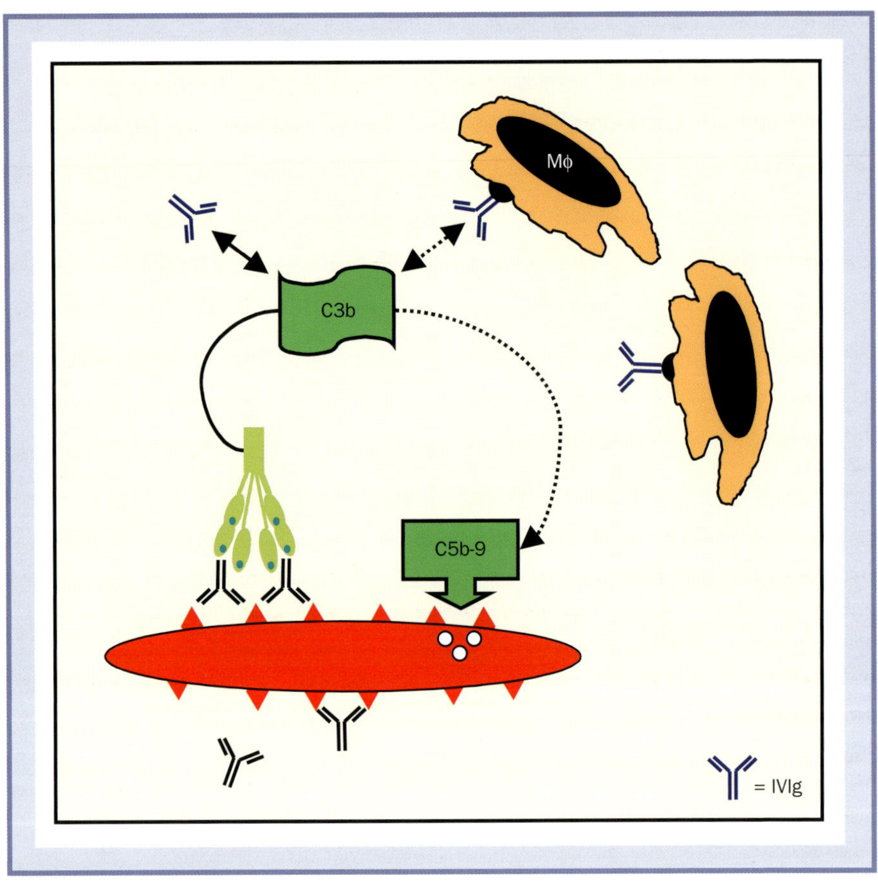



**Fig. 1.4**
*IVIg may act by neutralizing complement. By binding to C3b it may prevent the assembly of the C3 and C5 convertases and thereby block complement activation at an early step. Furthermore, IVIg may interfere with the formation of the terminal membrane attack complex (MAC, C5b-9).*

reconstituted with guinea pig C4. In normal guinea pigs shock could also be terminated by the intravenous administration of large doses of human γ-globulin prior to the injection of the anti-Forssman antibody. IVIg is capable of inhibiting cellular uptake of complement fragments C3 and C4, disrupting the formation and deposition of MAC[32] (Table 1.2).

## Interference with antibody-dependent cellular cytotoxicity

Macrophages exhibit pleotropic functions in the immune system and are crucial effector cells in many inflammatory disorders. They represent a cellular component of the innate immune system and, as such, do not express specific antigen receptors, such as B or T lymphocytes, but possess receptors for carbohydrates, and therefore can to some degree discriminate between 'self' and 'foreign' molecules. Moreover, they have receptors for antibodies and complement receptors. Opsonization ('coating') of pathogens with antibodies and/or complement will enhance macrophage activity. In some cases macrophages are able to destroy pathogens by phagocytosis without the need for T-cell activation. However, in many clinically important settings CD4[+] T cells are required to provide activating signals for macrophages. Once activated, macrophages can kill intracellular and ingested bacteria. Moreover, activated macrophages can also cause local tissue damage by the release of toxic oxygen free radicals and a host of other proinflammatory mediators.

IVIg may bind to Fc receptors on macrophages and thereby modulate their affinity by either saturating, altering or downregulating them (Figs 1.5 and 1.6). Inhibition of a host of macrophage functions, including phagocytosis, and the elaboration of an array of injurious molecules may be of key relevance to the therapeutic efficacy of IVIg in various inflammatory disorders. Recently, Samuelsson and co-workers demonstrated that antibody binding to the inhibitory Fc receptor, FcγRIIB, is important in modulating the anti-inflammatory activity of IVIg.[18] Saturation of Fc receptors on macrophages may also prevent the binding of autoantibodies which via their Fab fragments, could direct these phagocytic cells to their target antigens. Macrophages may thus be rendered unable to reach and damage structures in the target tissue.[33–35] The Fc region of the immunoglobulin mediates the effector properties of the molecule but not its immunologic specificity, which depends on its F(ab')2 fragment. When Imbach et al.[1] improved the platelet count in patients with idiopathic thrombocytopenic purpura with IVIg, blockade of Fc receptors was believed to be the major mechanism.

## Effects on T-cell activation

As indicated above, preparations of IVIg contain variable amounts of soluble CD4, CD8, major histocompatibility complex class 1 (MHC-I) and MHC-II molecules that could potentially interfere with the formation and function of the trimolecular complex of the T-cell receptor, autoantigenic peptide, and

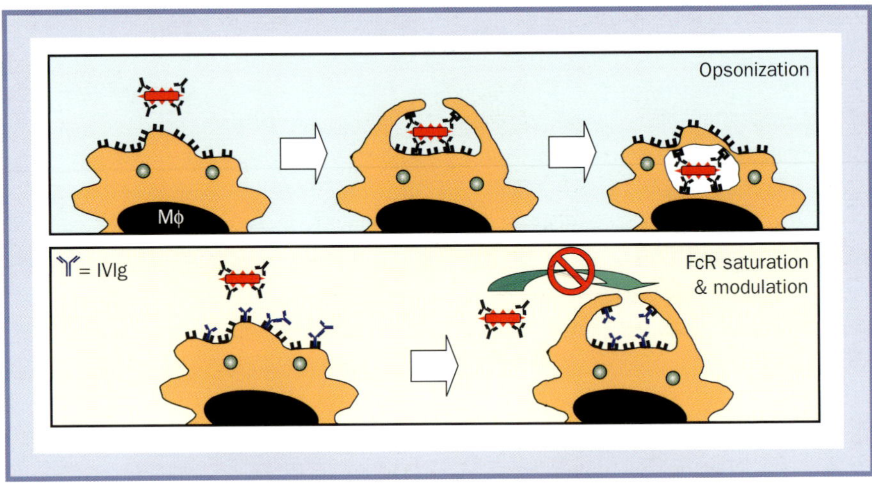



**Fig. 1.5**

*Fc receptors are important, among other functions, in triggering antibody-mediated cell activation. For example, foreign antigen covered by antibodies is more readily taken up by macrophages, a process called opsonization. IVIg may saturate Fc receptors or change their affinity and therefore intervene with autoantibody-mediated cellular activation.*

MHC molecules sometimes called the immunological synapse. Such interference could potentially inhibit autoreactive T lymphocytes. A similar effect could be mediated by antibodies against T-cell receptor Vβ chains, which have been detected in IVIg preparations[36] IVIg may also downregulate the expression of the accessory adhesion molecule lymphocyte function-associated antigen-1 (LFA-1) on activated T cells.[37] LFA-1 is one of the molecules critically involved in the interaction between T lymphocytes and antigen-presenting cells. Thus, IVIg may interfere with antigen presentation and T-cell activation. Moreover, Takei et al. were able to show that neutralizing antibodies to bacterial or viral superantigens, which may activate T cells non-specifically, are present in IVIg.[38]

## Restoration of a disturbed Th1/Th2 cytokine balance

Based on the expression of surface molecules, T lymphocytes can be differentiated into CD4[+] and CD8[+] cells. CD4[+] T cells usually act as helper T (Th) cells and recognize antigens presented by MHC class II molecules, whereas CD8[+] T cells are usually

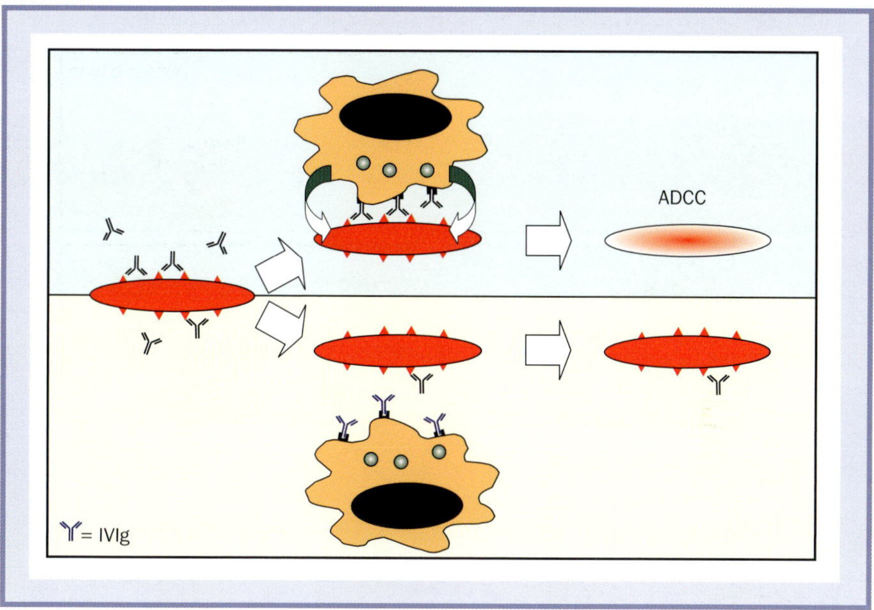



**Fig. 1.6**
*IVIg inhibits antibody-dependent cellular cytotoxicity (ADCC).*

cytotoxic and recognize antigens presented by MHC class I molecules. Once a naive CD4$^+$ T lymphocyte encounters a specific antigen on the surface of a professional antigen-presenting cell in the context of co-stimulatory molecules, the T cell becomes activated, proliferates, and differentiates into an effector Th lymphocyte. Three types of such effector Th cells are recognised: Th1 cells, manufacturing effector molecules that activate macrophages, Th2 cells generating B cell-activating effector molecules, and Th0 cells, from which both these functional classes derive, which secrete molecules characteristic of both Th1 and Th2 cells and may therefore have a distinct effector function. Interferon (IFN)-$\gamma$ is the signature cytokine of Th1 cells, which are important in phagocyte-mediated defence against infections. In contrast, Th2 populations produce interleukin (IL)-4 and IL-5 in response to helminths, parasites and allergic stimuli, resulting in downstream IgE production by B cells and eosinophil/mast cell-mediated immune reactions. Thus, effector T cells are critically involved in directing the effector functions of the adaptive immune response. The cytokines produced by the individual subclass of Th cells not only determine their effector function but also regulate the development and expansion of the respective subset. For example, IFN-γ, produced by Th1 cells, promotes further Th1 differentiation and inhibits the proliferation of Th2 cells. On the other hand, IL-4, secreted by Th2 lymphocytes, promotes Th2 differentiation, whereas IL-10, also produced by Th2 cells, inhibits the activation of Th1 lymphocytes. Thus, each Th subset amplifies itself and cross-regulates the reciprocal subset, and it is clear that the balance between Th1 and Th2 needs to be tightly controlled.

In various immune-mediated disorders a disturbed Th1/Th2 cytokine balance can be observed. IVIg has been implicated in redressing such a disturbance by supplying neutralizing antibodies that bind Th1 cytokines, cytokine antagonists and contaminating Th2 cytokines such as transforming growth factor-β.[39–44] *In vitro* studies have demonstrated that the addition of IVIg on the one hand suppresses the generation of Th1 cytokines, and on the other hand enhances the production of Th1 cytokine antagonists and Th2 cytokines by T lymphocytes.[45]

## Inhibition of cell adhesion

Vassilev and co-workers[46] recently reported that IVIg preparations contain antibodies directed to the Arg-Gly-Asp (RGD) motif, the attachment site of a number of adhesive extracellular matrix proteins, including ligands for β1, β3 and β5 integrins. This observation suggests that IVIg may affect the migration of immunocompetent cells from blood to the target tissues, potentially modifying local inflammatory responses (Fig. 1.7).

## Modulation of cellular proliferation and apoptosis

In order to control the massive expansion of cellular and soluble immune mediators certain mechanisms must operate with high fidelity to regulate the immune response. Once the target antigen has been eliminated, or infection resolved, the activated effector cells are no longer needed. The cessation of the antigenic stimulus prompts the cells to undergo programmed cell death, or *apoptosis.*[47]

IVIg has been shown to inhibit the proliferation of activated T and B lymphocytes,[48] and to induce apoptosis in leukaemic cells of lymphocyte and monocyte lineage, as well as CD40-activated normal B cells. A substantial suppression of proliferation of specifically activated T cells, in the absence

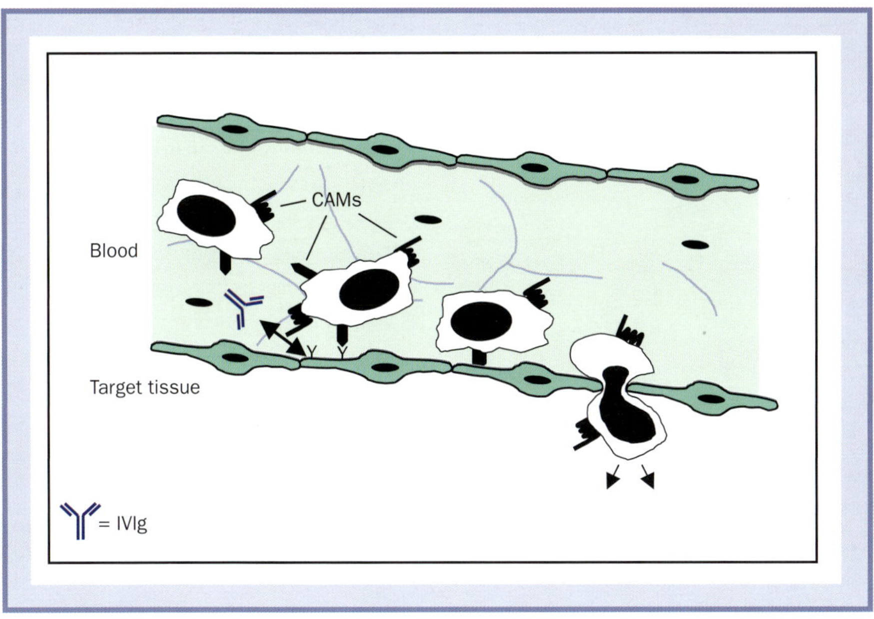



**Fig. 1.7**
*By interacting with adhesive extracellular matrix proteins IVIg may affect the migration of immunocompetent cells from blood to the target tissue.*

of caspase activation or DNA fragmentation, was found *in vitro* following treatment with IVIg. On the other hand, IVIg did not modulate the susceptibility of T cells to undergo CD95 (Fas/APO-1)-mediated apoptosis or the expression of apoptosis-blocking Bcl-2.[49] However, other studies revealed that IVIg induces apoptosis in activated CD95-positive mononuclear cells, exhibiting a striking increase in the expression of p21/WAF-1, suggesting G1 arrest as well as an upregulation of Bcl-2. It is conceivable, at least in theory, that IVIg may promote cell death in autoreactive T lymphocytes.[50]

In addition IVIg has been shown to contain antibodies that block Fas-dependent mechanisms, which have been shown to be involved in the therapeutic efficacy of IVIg in toxic epidermal necrolysis (TEN), preventing keratinocyte apoptosis.[51] Along similar lines, IVIg used in atopic dermatitis, and allergic contact dermatitis was demonstrated to inhibit keratinocyte apoptosis induced by activated T cells.[52] Taken together, these findings suggest that IVIg can alter cell cycle progression and modulate apoptosis.

## Effect on glucocorticoid receptor sensitivity

IVIg has been used as a glucocorticoid-sparing agent in a wide range of disorders in an attempt to avoid the multiple potential side effects of systemic corticosteroids, especially when used at high doses over prolonged periods. The combination of high-dose IVIg and corticosteroids is more effective than monotherapy in various immune-mediated disorders.[53–55] Spahn and co-workers showed that IVIg therapy was associated with increased glucocorticoid receptor (GC receptor) sensitivity, and that IVIg acted synergistically with corticosteroids in suppressing lymphocyte activation.[56] Thus, if prolonged immunosuppression is indicated for the treatment of a specific immune-mediated disorder, IVIg may be a safe and effective therapeutic option.[57] When IVIg is used adjunctively it is not clear what the most appropriate second-line agents are: these may vary with the condition being treated; however, the effects on GC receptor binding suggest a synergistic effect. More information regarding which agents synergize most effectively with IVIg are needed to aid rational prescribing and the most effective use of this scarce and expensive resource.

## Conclusion

Intravenous immunoglobulins have been shown to be efficacious in the treatment of numerous immune-mediated disorders. All preparations contain a vast range of antibody specificities in addition to other immunologically active molecules. Many potential mechanisms of action have been described though in many immune mediated disorders the exact mechanisms responsible for the observed benefits are not fully understood. Further studies are clearly warranted to elucidate new and important mechanisms of action of IVIg, and to better define dosage, timing and the most appropriate adjunctive agents in the establishment of evidence based treatment protocols. It is likely that a better understanding of the mechanisms of action of IVIg will also lead to an improved understanding of pathogenesis in the disease being studied.

## References


1. Imbach P, Barandun S, d'Apuzzo V et al. High-dose intravenous gammaglobulin for idiopathic thrombocytopenic purpura in childhood. *Lancet* 1981; **i**: 1228–31.

2. Carroll MC, Prodeus AP. Linkages of innate and adaptive immunity. *Curr Opin Immunol* 1998;**10**: 36–40.

3. Ochsenbein AF, Zinkernagel RM. Natural antibodies and complement link innate and acquired immunitiy. *Immunol Today* 2000; **21**: 624–30.

4. Edelman GM. Antibody structure and molecular immunology. *Science* 1979; **180**: 830–40.

5. Archelos JJ, Hartung H-P. Pathogenetic roles of autoantibodies in neurological diseases. *Trends Neurosci* 2000; **23**: 317–27.

6. Duhem C, Dicato MA, Ries F. Side-effects of intravenous immune globulins. *Clin Exp Immunol* 1994; **97** (Suppl 1): 79–83.

7. Ronda N, Kaveri SV, Kazatchkine MD. Treatment of autoimmune diseases with normal immunoglobulin through manipulation of the idiotypic network. *Clin Exp Immunol* 1993; **93** (Suppl 1): 14–15.

8. Rutter GH. Requirements for safety and quality of intravenous immunoglobulin G preparations. *J Neurol Neurosurg Psychiatry* 1994; **57** (Suppl): 2–5.

9. Kempf C, Jentsch P, Poirier B et al. Virus inactivation during production of intravenous immunoglobulin. *Transfusion* 1991; **31**: 423–7.

10. Kaveri SV, Dietrich G, Hurez V, Kazatchkine MD. Intravenous immunoglobulins (IVIg) in the treatment of autoimmune diseases. *Clin Exp Immunol* 1991; **86**: 192–8.

11. Morell A, Skvaril F. [Structure and biological properties of immunoglobulins and gamma-globulin preparations. II. Properties of gamma-globulin preparations]. *Schweiz Med Wschr* 1980; **110**: 80–5.

12. Burckhardt JJ, Gardi A, Oxelius VA et al. Immunoglobulin G subclass distribution in three human intravenous immunoglobulin preparations. *Vox Sang* 1989; **57**: 10–14.

13. Tokano Y, Umezawa Y, Okumura K. Determination of IgG subclasses of immunoglobulin preparations for intravenous injection and the problems involved. *Immunol Res* 1994; **13**: 56–60.

14. Grosse-Wilde H, Blasczyk R, Westhoff U. Soluble HLA class I and class II concentrations in commercial immunoglobulin preparations. *Tiss Antig* 1992; **39**: 74–7.

15. Blasczyk R, Westhoff U, Grosse-Wilde H. Soluble CD4, CD8, and HLA molecules in commercial immunoglobulin preparations. *Lancet* 1993; **341**: 789–90.

16. Stangel M, Hartung HP, Marx P, Gold R. Intravenous immunoglobulin treatment of neurological autoimmune diseases. *J Neurol Sci* 1998; **153**: 203–14.

17. Ratko TA, Burnett DA, Foulke GE, Matuszewski KA, Sacher RA. Recommendations for off-label use of intravenously administered immunoglobulin preparations. University Hospital Consortium Expert Panel for Off-Label Use of Polyvalent Intravenously Administered Immunoglobulin Preparations. *JAMA* 1995; **273**: 1865–70.

18. Samuelsson A, Towers TL, Ravetch JV. Anti-inflammatory activity of IVIG mediated through the inhibitory Fc receptor. *Science* 2001; **291**: 484–6.

19. Diegel ML, Rankin BM, Bolen JB, Dubois PM, Kiener PA. Cross-linking of Fc gamma receptor to surface immunoglobulin on B cells provides an inhibitory signal that closes the plasma membrane calcium channel. *J Biol Chem* 1994; **269**: 11409–16.

20. Kondo N, Kasahara K, Kameyama T et al. Intravenous immunoglobulins suppress immunoglobulin productions by suppressing Ca(2+)-dependent signal transduction through Fc gamma receptors in B lymphocytes. *Scand J Immunol* 1994; **40**: 37–42.

21. Zhuang Q, Mazer B. Inhibition of IgE production in vitro by intact and fragmented intravenous immunoglobulin. *J Allergy Clin Immunol* 2001; **108**: 229–34.

22. Kazatchkine MD, Dietrich G, Hurez V et al. V region-mediated selection of autoreactive repertoires by intravenous immunoglobulin (i.v.Ig). *Immunol Rev* 1994; **139**: 79–107.

23. Varela F, Andersson A, Dietrich G et al. Population dynamics of natural antibodies in normal and autoimmune individuals. *Proc Natl Acad Sci USA* 1991; **88**: 5917–21.

24. Noh G, Lozano F. Intravenous immune globulin effects on serum-soluble CD5 levels in atopic dermatitis. *Clin Exp Allergy* 2001; **31**: 1932–8.

25. Yu Z, Lennon VA. Mechanism of intravenous immune globulin therapy in antibody-mediated autoimmune diseases. *N Engl J Med* 1999; **340**: 227–8.

26. Tankersley DL, Preston MS, Finlayson JS. Immunoglobulin G dimer: an idiotype-anti-idiotype complex. *Mol Immunol* 1988; **25**: 41–8.

27. Dietrich G, Kazatchkine MD. Normal immunoglobulin G (IgG) for therapeutic use (intravenous Ig) contain antiidiotypic specificities against an immunodominant, disease-associated, cross-reactive idiotype of human anti-thyroglobulin autoantibodies. *J Clin Invest* 1990; **85**: 620–5.

28. Hurez V, Kazatchkine MD, Vassilev T et al. Pooled normal human polyspecific IgM contains neutralizing anti-idiotypes to IgG autoantibodies of autoimmune patients and protects from experimental autoimmune disease. *Blood* 1997; **90**: 4004–13.

29. Lacroix-Desmazes S, Kaveri SV, Mouthon L et al. Self-reactive antibodies (natural autoantibodies) in healthy individuals. *J Immunol Meth* 1998; **216**: 117–37.

30. Sultan Y, Kazatchkine MD, Maisonneuve P, Nydegger UE. Anti-idiotypic suppression of autoantibodies to factor VIII (antihaemophilic factor) by high-dose intravenous gammaglobulin. *Lancet* 1984; **ii**: 765–8.

31. May JE, Frank MM. Complement-mediated tissue damage: contribution of the classical and alternate complement pathways in the Forssman reaction. *J Immunol* 1972; **108**: 1517–25.

32. Lutz HU, Stammler P, Jelezarova E, Nater M, Spath PJ. High doses of immunoglobulin G attenuate immune aggregate-mediated complement activation by enhancing physiologic cleavage of C3b in C3bn-IgG complexes. *Blood* 1996; **88**: 184–93.

33. Hartung H-P, Gold R, Jung S. Local immune responses in the peripheral nervous system. In: Antel J, Birnbaum G, Hartung H-P, eds. *Clinical Neuroimmunology*. Malden, USA: Blackwell Science, 1998: 40–54.

34. Dalakas MC. Mechanism of action of intravenous immunoglobulin and therapeutic considerations in the treatment of autoimmune neurologic diseases. *Neurology* 1998; **51**(Suppl 5): S2–8.

35. Hartung H-P, Toyka KV, Griffin JW. Guillain–Barré syndrome and chronic inflammatory demyelinating polyradiculoneuropathy. In: Antel J, Birnbaum G, Hartung H-P, eds. *Clinical Neuroimmunology*. Malden, USA: Blackwell Science, 1998: 294–306.

36. Marchalonis JJ, Kaymaz H, Dedeoglu F, Schluter SF, Yocum DE, Edmundson AB. Human autoantibodies reactive with synthetic autoantigens from T-cell receptor beta chain. *Proc Natl Acad Sci USA* 1992; **89**: 3325–9.

37. Rigal D, Vermot-Desroches C, Heitz S, Bernaud J, Alfonsi F, Monier JC. Effects of intravenous immunoglobulins (IVIG) on peripheral blood B, NK, and T cell subpopulations in women with recurrent spontaneous abortions: specific effects on LFA-1 and CD56 molecules. *Clin Immunol Immunopathol* 1994; **71**: 309–14.

38. Takei S, Arora YK, Walker SM. Intravenous immunoglobulin contains specific antibodies inhibitory to activation of T cells by staphylococcal toxin superantigens. *J Clin Invest* 1993; **91**: 602–7.

39. Abe Y, Horiuchi A, Miyake M, Kimura S. Anti-cytokine nature of natural human immunoglobulin: one possible mechanism of the clinical effect of intravenous immunoglobulin therapy. *Immunol Rev* 1994; **139**: 5–19.

40. Aukrust P, Muller F, Svenson M, Nordoy I, Bendtzen K, Froland SS. Administration of intravenous immunoglobulin (IVIG) in vivo – down-regulatory effects on the IL-1 system. *Clin Exp Immunol* 1999; **115**: 136–43.

41. Kekow J, Reinhold D, Pap T, Ansorge S. Intravenous immunoglobulins and transforming growth factor beta. *Lancet* 1998; **351**: 184–5.

42. Pashov A, Dubey C, Kaveri SV et al. Normal immunoglobulin G protects against experimental allergic encephalomyelitis by inducing transferable T cell unresponsiveness to myelin basic protein. *Eur J Immunol* 1998; **28**: 1823–31.

43. Stangel M, Schumacher HC, Ruprecht K, Boegner F, Marx P. Immunoglobulins for intravenous use inhibit TNF alpha cytotoxicity in vitro. *Immunol Invest* 1997; **26**: 569–78.

44. Svenson M, Hansen MB, Bendtzen K. Binding of cytokines to pharmaceutically prepared human immunoglobulin. *J Clin Invest* 1993; **92**: 2533–9.

45. Pashov A, Bellon B, Kaveri SV, Kazatchkine MD. A shift in encephalitogenic T cell cytokine pattern is associated with suppression of EAE by intravenous immunoglobulins (IVIg). *Mult Scler* 1997; **3**: 153–6.

46. Vassilev TL, Kazatchkine MD, Van Huyen JP et al. Inhibition of cell adhesion by antibodies to Arg-Gly-Asp (RGD) in normal immunoglobulin for therapeutic use (intravenous immunoglobulin, IVIg). *Blood* 1999; **93**: 3624–31.

47. Gold R, Hartung HP, Lassmann H. T-cell apoptosis in autoimmune diseases: termination of inflammation in the nervous system and other sites with specialized immune-defense mechanisms. *Trends Neurosci* 1997; **20**: 399–404.

48. Amran D, Renz H, Lack G, Bradley K, Gelfand EW. Suppression of cytokine-dependent human T-cell proliferation by intravenous immunoglobulin. *Clin Immunol Immunopathol* 1994; **73**: 180–6.

49. Aktas O, Waiczies S, Grieger U, Wendling U, Zschenderlein R, Zipp F. Polyspecific immunoglobulins (IVIg) suppress proliferation of human (auto)antigen-specific T cells without inducing apoptosis. *J Neuroimmunol* 2001; **114**: 160–7.

50. Ekberg C, Nordstrom E, Skansen-Saphir U et al. Human polyspecific immunoglobulin for therapeutic use induces p21/WAF-1 and Bcl-2, which may be responsible for G1 arrest and long-term survival. *Hum Immunol* 2001; **62**: 215–27.

51. Viard I, Wehrli P, Bullani R et al. Inhibition of toxic epidermal necrolysis by blockade of CD95 with human intravenous immunoglobulin. *Science* 1998; **282**: 490–3.

52. Trautmann A, Akdis M, Schmid-Grendelmeier P et al. Targeting keratinocyte apoptosis in the treatment of atopic dermatitis and allergic contact dermatitis. *J Allergy Clin Immunol* 2001; **108**: 839–46.

53. Jolles S. High-dose intravenous immunoglobulin (hdIVIg) in the treatment of the autoimmune blistering disorders. *Clin Exp Immunol* 2002; **129**: 385–9.

54. Godeau B, Chevret S, Varet B et al. Intravenous immunoglobulin or high-dose methylprednisolone, with or without oral prednisone, for adults with untreated severe autoimmune thrombocytopenic purpura: a randomised, multicentre trial. *Lancet* 2002; **359**: 23–9.

55. Sami N, Qureshi A, Ahmed AR. Steroid sparing effect of intravenous immunoglobulin therapy in patients with pemphigus foliaceus. *Eur J Dermatol* 2002; **12**: 174–8.

56. Spahn JD, Leung DY, Chan MT, Szefler SJ, Gelfand EW. Mechanisms of glucocorticoid reduction in asthmatic subjects treated with intravenous immunoglobulin. *J Allergy Clin Immunol* 1999; **103**: 421–6.

57. Jolles S. A review of high-dose intravenous immunoglobulin treatment for atopic dermatitis. *Clin Exp Dermatol* 2002; **27**: 3–7.

# The role of high-dose intravenous  immunoglobulin in dermatomyositis

**Marinos C Dalakas**

**2**

DM: dermatomyositis; IBM: inclusion body myositis; ICAM: intercellular cell adhesion molecule; IVIg: intravenous immunoglobulin; LEMS: Lambert–Eaton myasthenic syndrome; LFA: lymphocyte function-associated antigen; MAC: membranolytic attack complex; MHC: major histocompatibility complex; MRC: Medical Research Council; mRNA: messenger RNA; N-CAM: neural cell adhesion molecule; NIH: National Institutes of Health; PM: polymyositis; TGF: transforming growth factor

## Introduction

The inflammatory myopathies are divided into three major and distinct subsets: polymyositis (PM), dermatomyositis (DM), and inclusion body myositis (IBM).[1–6] Although their cause is unknown, autoimmune mechanisms are implicated, as supported by their association with other putative or definite autoimmune diseases or viruses, the evidence for a

T cell-mediated myocytotoxicity or complement-mediated microangiopathy, and the presence of various autoantibodies.[1–6] This is also true for IBM, in spite of the coexistence of various degenerative features in these patients' muscle biopsies.[7,8]

Clinical experience indicates that patients with PM and DM respond to prednisone in some degree and for varying periods.[9–11] In some patients the response may be dramatic and, if prudently used, prednisone may have a long-lasting effect with minimal side-effects.[12] In other patients, however, the response is mild to moderate, and in still others the steroid-induced side-effects are severe, necessitating the use of other immunosuppressive drugs. Azathioprine, methotrexate, cyclosporin, cyclophosphamide and mycophenolate are commonly used immunosuppressants which offer a mild or, at the very best, a modest benefit, but with considerable toxicity after long-term use. Plasmapheresis is ineffective.[13] IBM is almost always unresponsive to steroids or other immunosuppressants. The need for more effective therapies and the encouraging results from pilot or uncontrolled studies[14–17] have prompted the need to examine the therapeutic efficacy of high-dose intravenous immunoglobulin (IVIg), an immunomodulating drug with prohibitive cost but minimal toxicity. This chapter summarizes the value of IVIg in DM based on controlled studies the authors performed at the National Institutes for Health (NIH). The role of IVIg in the other inflammatory myopathies will not be discussed here as it is beyond the scope of this book, and because these patients do not present to dermatologists. The accessibility of muscle biopsy tissues before and after therapy has also offered the opportunity to study the mechanism of action of IVIg and provide information useful in understanding how IVIg works, not only in inflammatory myopathies but also in other autoimmune neurological and dermatological disorders.

## IVIg in dermatomyositis

Dermatomyositis affects the skeletal muscles, resulting in proximal muscle weakness, and also the skin, causing a characteristic violaceous rash on the face, chest, knees, back and the knuckles of the fingers.[1–6] Dilated or infarcted capillaries at the bases of the fingernails are frequently present. The muscle biopsy shows endomysial inflammation which is predominantly perivascular or in the interfascicular septa and around, rather than within, the fascicles. The earliest lesion that precedes inflammation or structural changes in the muscle fibers is the deposition of the complement C5b–9 membranolytic attack complex (MAC) on the intramuscular capillaries.[1–6,18,19] This is followed by necrosis and a marked reduction in the number of capillaries per muscle fiber, especially in the perifascicular regions, resulting in ischemia and muscle fiber destruction which often resembles microinfarcts. Cytokines and adhesion molecules participate in the trafficking of sensitized lymphocytes and macrophages from the intramuscular blood vessels to the muscle fibers.[1-6] These molecules may be also responsible for the upregulation of the major histocompatibility complex (MHC) class I antigen expression on the muscle fibers, especially in the perifascicular regions, which are the areas most severely affected by the immunopathological process. Considering all the aforementioned immune mechanisms, if IVIg is effective in DM one may expect to see not only clinical benefit but also improvement in the muscle cytoarchitecture, downregulation of cytokines or adhesion molecules, effect on the complement activation and MAC formation, and improvement of the muscle microvasculature. Evidence that IVIg has an impressive effect in all these parameters is given below.

## Results of a controlled study

To assess the effect of IVIg in patients with DM a double-blind placebo-controlled study was conducted.[18] Patients incompletely responsive to various immunotherapeutic agents or those who had experienced significant side-effects from long-term steroid therapy were selected. A total of 15 patients (aged 18–55 years) with biopsy-proven treatment-resistant dermatomyositis were randomly assigned to receive IVIg (a total of 2 g/kg daily) or placebo, every month for 3 months, with the option of crossing over to the alternative therapy for 3 more months after a washout period of 1 month. The patients continued to receive prednisone at a mean daily dose (25 mg) that remained unchanged for 3 months before and after therapy. Clinical response was gauged by assessing changes in:

(a) muscle strength, using a modified MRC scale, a well-validated scale in the treatment of neuromuscular disorders;
(b) scores of neuromuscular symptoms that provide a picture of the daily living activities;
(c) the rash, using photography under the same lighting conditions.

Details of the methodology and scales have already been reported.[18] Further, a histological and immunopathological improvement was sought on the basis of quantitative histochemistry and immunopathology performed in repeated muscle biopsies.

Of the 15 patients, eight were assigned to IVIg and seven to placebo. Their mean scores at randomization and the mean disease duration in years were similar in both groups

(Table 2.1).[18] The patients randomized to IVIg had a significant improvement in the scores of muscle strength, from a mean of $76.6 \pm 5.7$ to $84.6 \pm 4.6$, and in the neuromuscular symptom scores, from a mean of $44 \pm 8.2$ to $51.4 \pm 6$. In contrast, the seven patients assigned to placebo did not change and their scores remained the same, from $78.6 \pm 6.3$ to $78.6 \pm 8.2$ and from $45.9 \pm 9.0$ to $45.7 \pm 11.3$, respectively (Table 2.1). The difference in scores between baseline and the end of treatment among IVIg and placebo-treated patients was significant ($P<0.018$ for the muscle strength and $P<0.035$ for the neuromuscular symptoms). With crossovers, a total of 12 patients received IVIg; of those, nine with severe disabilities had a major improvement (defined as more than 5 grades increase in the MRC scores) reaching nearly normal function, two had mild improvement and one had no change (Table 2.2). The mean muscle strength scores in these nine patients increased from $74.5 \pm 4.9$ to $84.7 \pm 4.5$. Their neuromuscular symptoms also improved significantly, from $38.6 \pm 5.9$ to $51 \pm 8.0$.[19] The statistically significant improvements in muscle strength, expressed as MRC and neuromuscular symptom scores, were functionally impressive for individual patients, some of whom were wheelchair bound before therapy and who walked independently or regained full strength after 3 months of IVIg. Of 11 placebo-treated patients, none had major improvement, three had mild improvement, three had no change in their condition, and five worsened (Table 2.2). Even though this is a

**Table 2.1**

*Response to IVIg in a placebo-controlled study of patients with dermatomyositis. Values are mean manual muscle strength (MRC) scores and mean neuromuscular symptom (NS) scores*

| Therapy | Mean duration of disease (years) | Pretreatment | | After treatment* | |
| --- | --- | --- | --- | --- | --- |
| | | MRC | NS | MRC | NS |
| IVIg (n = 8) | 3.9 | $76.6 \pm 5.7$ | $44.1 \pm 8.2$ | $84.6 \pm 4.6^{\dagger}$ | $51.4 \pm 6.0^{\ddagger}$ |
| Placebo (n = 7) | 3.8 | $78.6 \pm 6.3$ | $45.9 \pm 9.0$ | $78.6 \pm 8.2$ | $45.7 \pm 11.3$ |

*Response to IVIg or placebo was measured after 3 months of treatment and before crossover to the alternative therapy, the effect of which is shown in Fig. 2.1 (see text for details).
$^{\dagger}P = 0.018$ (Wilcoxon) for comparison with placebo value.
$^{\ddagger}P = 0.035$ (Wilcoxon) for comparison with placebo value.

**Table 2.2**
*Response to IVIg in a placebo-controlled study of patients with dermatomyositis, including a crossover phase*

| Response | Placebo (n = 11) | IVIg (n = 12) |
|---|---|---|
| Major improvement* | 0 | 9 |
| Mild improvement[†] | 3 | 2 |
| No change | 3 | 1 |
| Deterioration | 5 | 0 |

*Defined as a more than 5-grade increase in both the total MRC score and the total neuromuscular symptom score.
[†]Defined as an increase of 2–5 grades in the total MRC score and the total neuromuscular symptom score.

small series, the results were not only statistically significant but clinically impressive.

The improvement became noticeable about 15 days after the first IVIg infusion and it was clear and definitive after the second. Only two of the responders reached their peak after the second infusion; the rest peaked between the second and third infusions. Eight patients had marked improvement of the active violaceous rash, or the chronic scaly eruptions on their knuckles, which often preceded or coincided with the improvement of muscle strength. Serum creatine kinase levels, elevated up to 10-fold in seven of the IVIg-treated patients, fell by 50% after the first infusion and decreased further or normalized by the second infusion. Creatine kinase levels remained elevated, were unchanged, or increased during placebo, and returned to baseline 6–10 weeks after the

IVIg-treated patients crossed over to placebo or the IVIg infusions were stopped. Overall, the patients who noted a major improvement felt that IVIg had a serious impact on their daily activities, without troublesome adverse effects.

In subsequent open-labeled infusions the benefit of IVIg was also documented in more than 30 patients treated by the author's group or under our supervision in several institutions. The improvement was also documented in one of the open-label-treated patients using quantitative muscle strength testing – the maximal voluntary isometric contractions method – which measures changes in muscle strength in newtons (N). In this patient, the scores improved from 202 N at baseline to 358 N after the third infusion. Before therapy she used a cane to walk, but became able to exercise on parallel bars after two IVIg infusions.[19]

## Role of IVIg in maintaining response

The improvement in strength is usually short-lived, lasting not more than 4–8 weeks. Most of the original patients from this study whose follow-up data are available continue to receive IVIg and respond to a variable degree. Some patients need IVIg less frequently and continue to maintain their improvement in conjunction with low-dose steroids; two patients who were wheelchair bound prior to therapy and received IVIg for 2 years have maintained normal strength without any drugs for 3–5 years; others need IVIg every 3–4 weeks to maintain an excellent response, and some others continue to improve on 4–6-week regimens, but the improvement is not as impressive as initially, presumably because of further progression of the disease or a diminished response to IVIg therapy. In several patients it was possible to lower the prednisone dose and keep it at a low maintenance level. It is the author's experience that low-dose prednisone is helpful and appears to enhance the benefit of IVIg. It was also noted that some patients who had become unresponsive to steroids responded again to prednisone after a few IVIg infusions. The phenomenon of restoring responsiveness to steroids is an interesting one and needs to be further studied, not only in DM but also in chronic inflammatory demyelinating polyneuropathy, where it has been also noted (author's unpublished observations). A possible explanation for this synergistic effect is the recent evidence that IVIg enhances glucocorticoid receptor-binding affinity.[20]

## How IVIg exerts its action: studies on repeated muscle biopsies and on post-IVIg sera

In patients who showed major improvement, repeat open muscle biopsies on the biceps muscle opposite the one used for the pretreatment biopsy were performed 15 days after the last IVIg infusion. Before the code was broken, the pretreatment biopsies were processed for muscle enzyme histochemistry and immunocytochemistry in an immunoperoxidase technique, using antibodies against MHC-I, ICAM-I, Leu-19 (to assess the regenerating muscle fibers) and various lymphocyte subsets[15] and TGF-β-protein and mRNA. Further, the capillaries were visualized by immunofluorescence and immunoperoxidase staining, using the lectin *Ulex europaeus*, which stains the capillary endothelial cells.[18,19] In five randomly selected perifascicular regions at a low original ($\times$40) magnification, each region corresponding to a large $6.4 \times 10^4$ μm$^2$ surface area, the number of capillaries and their diameter were counted, as well as the number of muscle fibers and their diameter, and the ratio of muscle fiber to capillaries was calculated (Table 2.3 and Fig. 2.1). The biopsy measurements following treatment were compared not only with the pretreatment biopsies but also with five biopsies from patients with limb-girdle dystrophies, who served as disease controls.

A marked improvement in muscle histology was noted in the repeat biopsies compared with the pre-IVIg biopsies. As shown in Table 2.3, the mean number of muscle fibers counted in the five regions decreased as a result of an increase in the muscle fiber diameter, from a mean of $54.0 \pm 11\,\mu m$ to $71.0 \pm 15\,\mu m$ ($P < 0.04$). The mean number of capillaries increased and their mean diameter decreased from $11.0 \pm 3\,\mu m$ to $7.4 \pm 2\,\mu m$ (normal, $6.5 \pm 0.1\,\mu m$) ($P < 0.01$) (Table 2.3). The mean ratio of muscle fibers to capillaries also decreased from 3.4 to 1.5 (normal 1.2) and normalized in three patients (Table 2.3).

Among the main immunological markers on the repeat biopsy was the downregulation of the MHC-I molecule, which was markedly expressed in the pretreatment biopsy in the perifascicular regions (Fig. 2.2). In addition, ICAM-I expression on the surface of some muscle fibers and on the blood vessels was suppressed after IVIg therapy.[18] Because ICAM-I, the ligand for LFA-I, was overexpressed on the endothelial cells before therapy, its IVIg-induced downregulation probably had an effect on the exit of activated T cells from the capillaries towards the muscle fibers, and might have been responsible for the reduction of inflammatory cells noted in

**Table 2.3**

*Effect of IVIg on histological characteristics in the muscles of patients with dermatomyositis*

| | Pretreatment (n = 5) | After treatment (n = 5) |
|---|---|---|
| Muscle fibers* | 34.2±2 | 24.8±8 |
| Muscle fiber diameter (μm) | 54 ± 11 | 71±15[†] |
| Capillaries* | 13.5±3 | 18.2 6 4.8 (normal 19.7±6.7) |
| Capillary diameter (μm) | 11.0±2.8 | 7.4±2[‡] (normal 6.5±0.01) |
| Muscle fiber : capillaries | 3.4 | 1.54 (normal 1.2) |

*Mean number of muscle fibers or capillaries in five randomly selected perifascicular regions at a low, original (×40) magnification, each region corresponding to a $6.4 \times 10^4\ \mu m^2$ surface area (see text for details).
[†]P = 0.04 (ANOVA) for comparison with pretreatment value.
[‡]P = 0.01 (ANOVA) for comparison with pretreatment value.

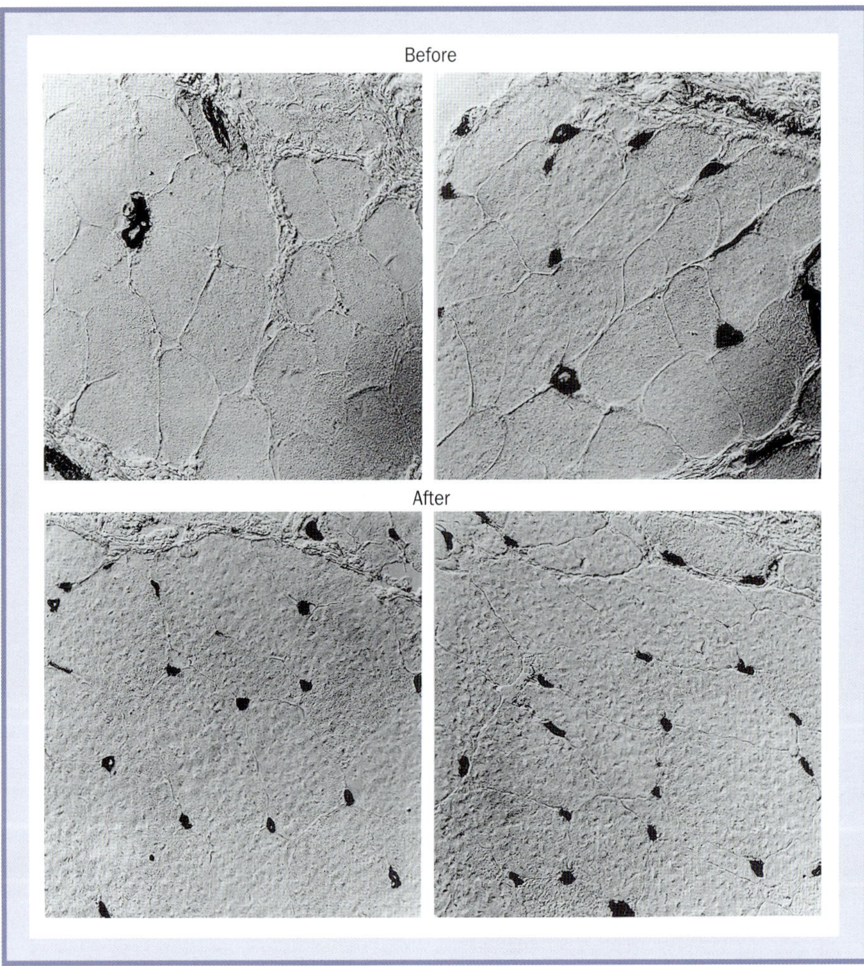



**Fig. 2.1**
*Cross-section of representative muscle areas before therapy (top panels) and after therapy (lower panels) stained for Ulex europaeus, which identifies the endothelial cells (see quantification of capillaries in Table 2.3). An increase in the number of capillaries and reduction in fiber diameter is shown after therapy (lower panels). The same magnification is used for both.*

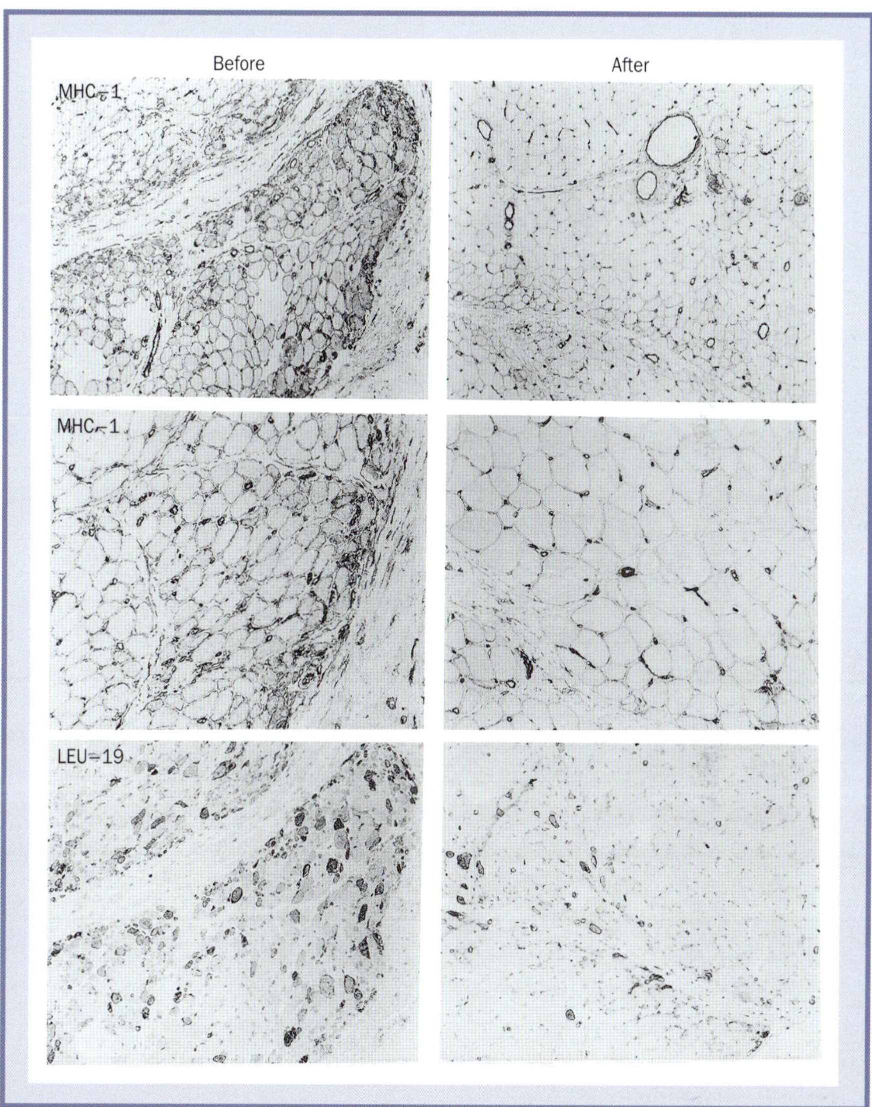



**Fig. 2.2**

*Cross-section of muscle biopsies stained for MHC-I (top and middle figure) and for Leu-19 (low figure) before (left) and after IVIg therapy (right) shows the marked suppression of MHC-I expression and the downregulation of Leu-19-positive fibers. The increase in the diameter of the muscle fibers, especially in the periphery, is prominent after therapy. The perivascular inflammatory responses seen before, as MHC-positive cells, improved after therapy. Two MHC-I figures are shown (top and middle) at different magnifications.*

the repeat biopsies. Another effect of IVIg was on TGF-β expression. TGF-β is a pleiotropic cytokine which, when in excess, induces chronic inflammation and fibrosis. In the tissues of DM patients TGF-β is upregulated at both the protein and the mRNA level.[21] After IVIg, the repeat muscle biopsies revealed an impressive downregulation of TGF-β and TGF-β mRNA. Interestingly, this effect was not observed in five repeat muscle biopsies from patients with inclusion body myositis who did not respond to IVIg.[20]

The most remarkable improvement with regard to the immunopathogenetic mechanism of DM was the IVIg-induced interception of the formation and intramuscular deposition of the membranolytic attack complex, the lytic component of the complement pathway. In the repeat muscle biopsies the C3bNEO (neoantigen), which is immune-complex specific, and the MAC could not be detected in the endomysial capillaries.[22–24] Further, in an assay system of *in vitro* sensitized erythrocytes the consumption of C3 uptake by the patients' sera was suppressed after IVIg, compared with the pretreatment sera.[22] As discussed in the mechanism of action of IVIg,[25,26] IVIg inhibited the incorporation of C3 into the C5 convertase assembly, prevented the formation of C3bNEO[25] and intercepted the formation and deposition of MAC on the endomysial capillaries. Consequently, IVIg allowed

neovascularization and the reversal of the ischemic process, as demonstrated by the normalization of the capillaries and the muscle fiber diameter in the repeat muscle biopsies (see Figs 2.1 and 2.2).

The effect of IVIg in intercepting the formation and deposition of MAC in target tissues may be also relevant to other IVIg-responsive diseases in which tissue damage is mediated by complement activation and MAC deposition. For example, MAC deposition mediates the destruction not only of the capillaries in DM but also of the myelin sheath in Guillain–Barré syndrome and the acetylcholine receptors in myasthenia gravis.

# References


1. Dalakas MC. Polymyositis, dermatomyositis, and inclusion-body myositis. *N Engl J Med* 1991; **325**: 1487–98.

2. Engel AG, Hohlfeld R, Banker BQ. The polymyositis and dermatomyositis syndrome. In: Engel AG, Franzini-Armstrong C, eds. *Myology.* New York: McGraw-Hill, 1994: 1335–83.

3. Karpati G, Carpenter S. Pathology of the inflammatory myopathies. In: Mastaglia FL, ed. *Baillière's Clinical Neurology.* London: WB Saunders, 1993: 527–56.

4. Dalakas MC. Immunopathogenesis of inflammatory myopathies. *Ann Neurol* 1995; **37**: 74–86.

5. Dalakas MC. Immunopathogenesis of inflammatory myopathies. In: Antel JP, Birnbaum G, Hartung HP, eds. *Clinical*

*Neuroimmunology.* Oxford: Blackwell Science, 1998: 374–84.

6. Sivakumar K, Dalakas MC. Inclusion body myositis and myopathies. *Curr Opin Neurol* 1997; **10:** 413–20.

7. Koffman BM, Sivakumar K, Simonis T et al. HLA allele distribution distinguishes sporadic inclusion body myositis from hereditary inclusion body myopathies. *J Neuroimmunol* 1998; **84:** 139–42.

8. Koffman BM, Rugiero M, Dalakas MC. Autoimmune diseases and autoantibodies associated with sporadic inclusion body myositis. *Muscle Nerve* 1998; **21:** 115–17.

9. Dalakas MC. How to diagnose and treat the inflammatory myopathies. *Semin Neurol* 1994; **14:** 137–45.

10. Dalakas MC. The treatment of polymyositis, dermatomyositis and inclusion body myositis. In: Johnson RT, Griffin JW, eds. *Current Therapy in Neurology.* St Louis: Mosby/Year Book, 1996: 407–12.

11. Dalakas MC. Polymyositis, dermatomyositis and inclusion body myositis. In: Kassirer JP, Greene HL, eds. *Current Therapy in Adult Medicine.* St Louis: Mosby/Year Book, 1997: 1434–9.

12. Dalakas MC. Treatment of polymyositis and dermatomyositis. *Curr Opin Rheumatol* 1989; **1:** 443–9.

13. Miller FW, Leitman SF, Cronin ME et al. Controlled trial of plasma exchange and leukopheresis in polymyositis and dermatomyositis. *N Engl J Med* 1992; **326:** 1380–4.

14. Cherin P, Herson S, Wechsler B et al. Efficacy of intravenous immunoglobulin therapy in chronic refractory polymyositis and dermatomyositis. An open study with 20 adult patients. *Am J Med* 1991; **91:** 162–8.

15. Lang B, Laxer RM, Murphy G et al. Treatment of dermatomyositis with intravenous immunoglobulin. *Am J Med* 1991; **91:** 169–72.

16. Jan S, Beretta S, Moggio M et al. High-dose intravenous human immunoglobulin in polymyositis resistant to treatment. *J Neurol Neurosurg Psychiatry* 1992; **55:** 60–4.

17. Soueidan SA, Dalakas MC. Treatment of inclusion-body myositis with high-dose intravenous immunoglobulin. *Neurology* 1993; **43:** 876–9.

18. Dalakas MC, Illa I, Dambrosia JM et al. A controlled trial of high-dose intravenous immunoglobulin infusions as treatment for dermatomyositis. *N Engl J Med* 1993; **329:** 1993–2000.

19. Dalakas MC. Intravenous immune globulin for dermatomyositis. *N Engl J Med* 1994; **330:** 1392–3.

20. Spahn JD, Leung DY, Chan MT et al. Mechanisms of glucocorticoid reduction in asthmatic subjects treated with intravenous immunoglobulin. *J Allergy Clin Immunol* 1999; **103:** 421–6.

21. Amemiya K, Semino-Mora C, Granger RP, Dalakas MC. Down regulation of TGF-$\beta_1$, mRNA and protein in the muscle of patients with inflammatory myopathy after treatment with high-dose intravenous immunoglobulin. *Clin Immunol* 2000; **94:** 99–104.

22. Dalakas MC. Experience with IVIg in the treatment of inflammatory myopathies. In: Kazatchkine L, Morel M, eds. *Intravenous Immunoglobulin Research and Therapy.* New York: Parthenon, 1996: 275–84.

23. Basta M, Dalakas MC. High-dose intravenous

immunoglobulin exerts its beneficial effect in patients with dermatomyositis by blocking endomysial deposition of activated complement fragments. *J Clin Invest* 1994; **94**: 1729–35.

24. Dalakas MC. Clinical relevance of IVIg in the modulation of the complement-mediated tissue damage: implications in dermatomyositis, Guillain–Barré syndrome and myasthenia gravis. In: Kazatchkine L, Morel M, eds. *Intravenous Immunoglobulin Research and Therapy.* New York: Parthenon, 1996: 89–93.

25. Dalakas MC. Mechanism of action of intravenous immunoglobulin and therapeutic considerations in the treatment of autoimmune neurologic diseases. *Neurology* 1998; **51** (Suppl 5): S2–S8.

26. Dalakas MC. Intravenous immunoglobulin in the treatment of autoimmune neuromuscular diseases: present status and practical therapeutic guidelines. *Muscle Nerve* 1999; **22**: 1479–97.

# Chronic urticaria

**Brigid F O'Donnell**

**Brigid F O'Donnell**

---

ANCA, antineutrophil cytoplasmic antibody; IVIg, intravenous immunoglobulins

---

## Introduction

Urticaria, derived from the Latin *urere*, to burn, describes an eruption of transient, circumscribed cutaneous swellings. The wheal or hive, an oedematous, erythematous papule or plaque, is the characteristic lesion in urticaria and is almost invariably itchy.[1] Angio-oedema is considered part of the same disease process as urticaria, but involves deeper tissues.[2] The swellings of angio-oedema are subcutaneous and usually also involve the mucous membranes, although they can occur anywhere on the body. Itching is variable and the swellings disappear in 24–72 hours. Angio-oedema may occur alone (11%), in combination with urticaria (49%), or urticaria may occur alone (40%).[2]

## Chronic urticaria and chronic 'idiopathic' urticaria

Strictly, the term 'chronic urticaria' should embrace all

urticarial eruptions lasting longer than the arbitrary 6–8 weeks and would include the various physical urticarias and drug-, food- or infection-related urticaria. However, many use the term chronic urticaria synonymously with chronic 'idiopathic' urticaria and refer to the particular physical urticaria – for example cold or cholinergic urticaria – by name. Chronic 'idiopathic' urticaria is, frustratingly, the most prevalent form of the disease accounting for 70–79% of those who attend hospital clinics with urticaria.[2,3] The term 'idiopathic' is no longer satisfactory,[4] as evidence is accumulating that a proportion of patients previously labelled as having chronic 'idiopathic' urticaria, have in fact 'autoimmune' urticaria.[5,6] The spectrum and heterogeneous nature of chronic urticaria has recently been comprehensively reviewed.[7]

## Clinical features

In chronic urticaria short-lived, oedematous and red cutaneous swellings (wheals) (Fig. 3.1a, b) sometimes with central clearing, continue to develop over a period of 6 weeks or longer.[8,9] Individual lesions, which are usually intensely itchy, last less than 24 hours and vary from red wheals and papules to larger plaques, which may be discoid, annular, or have a geographic configuration. Wheals range in size from 1 to 2 mm in diameter (micropapular urticaria) to lesions as large as 50 cm.[1] There are no associated epidermal changes and excoriation is exceptional,[10] as patients tend to rub rather than scratch. Unpredictable crops of wheals, due to local transient dermal oedema and vasodilatation, appear suddenly and resolve completely in 12–24 hours. However, fresh lesions may continue to appear almost indefinitely, and there is a tendency for wheals to develop at night.[9,10]

Some patients experience a prodromal phase lasting from a few hours to 1 or 2 days, associated with anorexia, malaise, headache and fever.[9] Systemic symptoms, including nausea, diarrhoea, abdominal pain, indigestion, joint pain, joint swelling,[11] depression, lassitude, fatigue, aching, shivering and flushing, are common during severe attacks.[12]

Chronic urticaria with or without angio-oedema may occur at any age, but most frequently develops during the third and fourth decades of life and is commoner in females.[10] Champion et al.[2] predicted that of patients with urticaria only, 50% will still have active urticaria at 6 months and more than 20% will still have active disease 20 years later. The prognosis is worse for those with both urticaria and angio-oedema.[2]

Chronic urticaria causes distress, discomfort and deterioration in the quality of life.[13] Using the Nottingham Health Profile as an index of day-to-day wellbeing, patients with chronic urticaria were compared with a cohort of patients with ischaemic heart

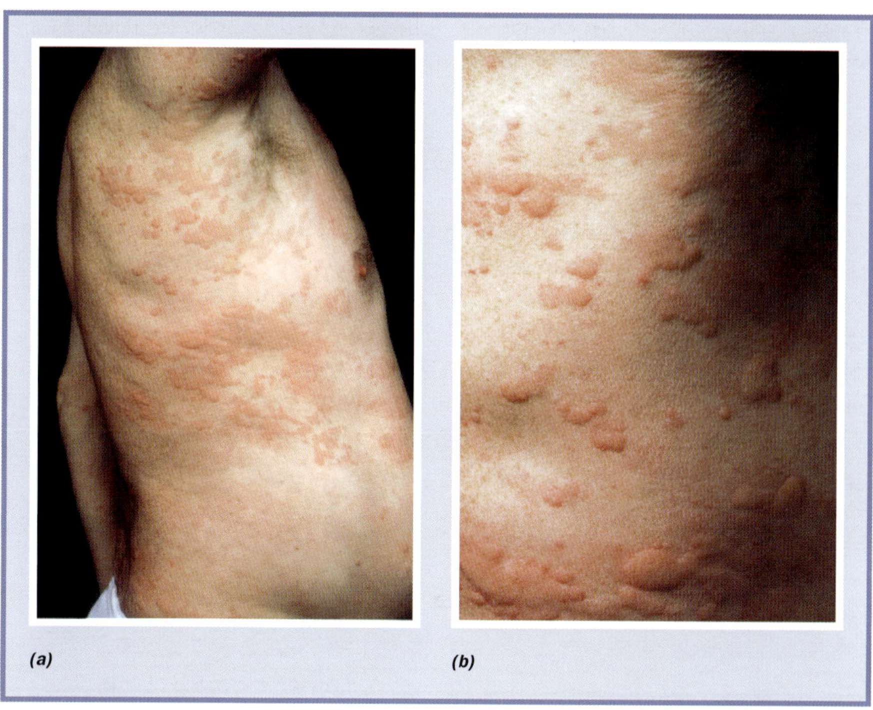

**Fig. 3.1a, b**
*(a) Urticarial wheals on the lateral aspect of the trunk. (b) Close-up view to emphasize the oedematous nature of individual wheals.*

disease. The two groups showed similar scores for problems with energy, social isolation and emotional upset. Limitation of mobility and pain were more severe in those with heart disease, but sleep disruption was a greater problem in the patients with urticaria.[13]

## Pathogenesis

The central role of histamine in producing the early, short-lived wheal-and-flare in urticaria has been recognized for many years.

### *The late-phase reaction*

In addition to the immediate, fleeting wheal-and-flare reaction that occurs following the introduction of allergen into the skin of sensitive humans, an indurated, tender, pruritic and erythematous swelling may develop 2–4 hours later and last 24–48 hours.[14,15] This late-phase reaction requires higher concentrations of allergen than are required for the immediate reaction, and can also be elicited by heterologous anti-IgE sera and by mast cell-activating agents such as compound 48/80. Histamine will not produce this effect and the late-phase cutaneous response seems dependent on mast cell activation.[15,16] The mediators in late-phase reactions, which have not yet been precisely identified, have chemotactic properties, recruiting inflammatory cells – initially neutrophils, and later mononuclear cells – from the blood into the tissue. The cells can secrete additional chemotactic and vasoactive mediators to amplify the reaction and maintain or increase whealing.[17]

## The cutaneous mast cell

Cutaneous mast cells are normally present in a perivascular distribution in the dermis and subcutaneous tissue[18] and are the primary effector cell type in urticaria and angio-oedema.[19] However, the finding of a 10-fold increase in the number of mast cells in the wheals of chronic idiopathic urticaria[20] has recently been questioned. Samples of lesional ($n=11$) and non-lesional ($n=9$) skin from patients were compared with site-matched skin from healthy controls ($n=10$).[21] Using a double-labelling immunohistochemical technique with specific monoclonal antibodies

to mast cell tryptase and chymase, Smith et al.[21] showed that there was no significant difference in mast cell numbers in the three sites tested. In both patients and controls more than 99% of cutaneous mast cells contained tryptase and chymase.[21]

Typically, mast cells are activated by cross-linking of the high-affinity receptor for IgE, but non-immunologic activation of mast cells occurs through direct degranulation (codeine), perturbation of arachidonic acid metabolism (aspirin), physical stimuli and idiosyncratic reactions.[19]

## Mast cell mediators

### Histamine

Regardless of whether the number of mast cells in urticaria is increased or unchanged, an increase in histamine level in suction blister fluid,[22] and in skin biopsy samples has been demonstrated,[23] and patients with urticaria show a prolonged skin whealing response to histamine compared to normal subjects.[24]

### Other mast cell mediators

In addition to histamine, human skin mast cells are capable of generating a variety of preformed (within mast cell granules) and newly synthesized (derived from the phospholipid cell membrane) mediators. These mediators, which include prostaglandin

D$_2$, leukotriene C$_4$, leukotriene B$_4$, heparin, interleukin-3, interleukin-5, interleukin-8, platelet-activating factor, granulocyte–macrophage colony-stimulating factor and tumour necrosis factor α, have multiple biological effects.[25]

Following degranulation, the various proinflammatory mediators have potential effects on inflammatory cells and the microvasculature, thereby extending the inflammatory response. However, the relative importance and the role(s) of the various mediators, apart from histamine, in the pathogenesis of chronic urticaria, are unclear.

## Histamine-releasing factor

Histamine-releasing factor, thought to represent cytokines, has been found in the blister fluid of lesional skin in chronic urticaria in significantly higher quantities than in non-lesional skin and the skin of controls.[26] Macrophage chemotactic protein-1, RANTES, and macrophage inflammatory protein-1α, are potent direct secretagogues for human basophils and interleukin-3, interleukin-5 and granulocyte–macrophage colony-stimulating factor are priming factors for the potentiation of mediator release from basophils.[27] These cytokines may play a role in the recruitment of inflammatory cells in the late-phase reaction. However, these cytokines or chemokines do not play a significant role in priming or stimulating skin mast cells.[27]

## Histamine-releasing activity and histamine-releasing autoantibodies

Grattan et al.[28,29] demonstrated the presence of a transferable factor in the sera of some patients during an active phase of chronic urticaria, by autologous intradermal serum tests. A wheal-and-flare response following the intradermal injection of autologous serum was shown in 7 of 12[28] and 8 of 16[29] patients tested. The serological mediator was not demonstrable in control subjects and no longer demonstrable during clinical remission, and was therefore of probable functional significance.[28] In a subsequent larger study, 20 of 25 patients had a positive autologous intradermal serum test.[12] Sera from 14 of these patients elicited histamine release from the basophil leukocytes of healthy donors, but sera from none of 10 healthy and five dermographic control subjects showed evidence of *in vivo* or *in vitro* histamine-releasing activity. Ultrafiltration of the patient sera showed that whealing was confined to ultrafiltered serum fractions > 100 kDa in all of nine patients tested. IgG, purified from the sera by affinity chromatography, retained the ability to release histamine from the basophil leukocytes of healthy donors. Functional studies using passive sensitization with myeloma IgE, desensitization with anti-IgE in the absence of calcium, and lactic acid stripping of donor basophils to remove bound IgE, followed by resensitization with IgE, suggested that the histamine-releasing autoantibody had the properties of anti-IgE.[12]

However, the ability of some serum samples to induce histamine release from the basophils of a blood donor with a low serum IgE suggested the presence of other, non-IgE-dependent histamine-releasing factors.[30] Using the mouse monoclonal antibody 6F7, which interacts with and cross-links adjacent IgE-binding sites on the α subunit of the high-affinity receptor (FcεRIα) as a positive control, four patients whose sera induced the substantial release of histamine from the basophils of a low-IgE donor and negligible release from the basophils of a high-IgE donor, were selected for study. Their histamine-releasing activity was competitive with IgE, as it was blocked by passive sensitization with myeloma IgE and subsequently restored by removing it. Serum IgG was isolated from each patient and all IgG fractions showed histamine-releasing activity, with dilution curves similar to those of whole serum and the IgE-competitive anti-FcεRIα monoclonal antibody, 6F7. To prove a direct interaction between the autoantibody and the high-affinity IgE receptor, the effect of incubation of basophils from a low-IgE donor with a recombinant preparation of the soluble extracellular domain of the α subunit of the high-affinity IgE receptor (sFcεRIα) on histamine-releasing activity was studied. As anticipated, the results showed an almost complete abolition of histamine release,

thereby substantiating the locus of binding of these patients' IgG on the α subunit of FcεRI.

The ability of some patients' sera to release histamine from the basophil leukocytes of both a low- and a high-IgE donor, resembling the non-IgE competitive monoclonal antibody 29C6, suggests that they may have antibodies reacting with the non-IgE-binding domain of FcεRIα, or a mixture of anti-FcεRIα antibodies of different specificities.[31] Thus, there are at least three types of histamine-releasing autoantibody, anti-IgE, anti-FcεRIα (IgE competitive) and anti-FcεRIα (non-IgE competitive) which may occur separately or together. The relative frequencies of the types of histamine-releasing autoantibody have yet to be established in larger populations. The presence anti-FcεRI antibodies in a third of patients with chronic urticaria has been confirmed by Stingl's group using immunoblotting and immunoprecipitation, and they have also confirmed that these autoantibodies are functional.[32] In retrospect, the basophilic leukopenia reported by Rorsman in certain types of urticaria,[33] was an early indicator of the presence of circulating degranulating factor(s). More recent work by Grattan et al.[12] has confirmed the reduction in stainable, peripheral blood basophils per $mm^3$ in 14 patients with chronic urticaria ($7.9 \pm 2.0$, mean $\pm$ SEM) compared to healthy controls ($39.6 \pm 4.4$, mean $\pm$ SEM, $P < 0.001$).[12]

# Chronic urticaria – an autoimmune disease

The criteria for the diagnosis of an autoimmune disease were modelled on Koch's postulates.[34] An update of these criteria suggests that direct, indirect and circumstantial evidence may be marshalled to establish that a human disease is actually autoimmune in origin.[35,36] In a proportion of patients with chronic urticaria, the identification of autoantibodies to the high-affinity IgE receptor,[30] the reproduction of the wheal by the injection of autologous serum, the ability of patient sera to release histamine from the basophil leukocytes of healthy donors *in vitro*, and the inverse correlation with blood basophil count and histamine content, support the concept that in these cases chronic urticaria is an autoimmune phenomenon. Positive passive transfer has also been reported.[6] Study of HLA class II associations in chronic urticaria showed a striking increased frequency of HLA DR4 (DRB1*04) and its associated allele DQ8 (DQB1*0302) in patients with chronic urticaria compared with the control population ($P = 2 \times 10^{-5}$ and $P = 2 \times 10^{-4}$, respectively).[37] The positive association with DR4 was particularly striking in patients whose serum showed *in vivo* and *in vitro* histamine-releasing activity ($P = 3.6 \times 10^{-6}$).[37]

# Chronic urticaria – three disease subsets

During active phases of chronic urticaria the primary cutaneous lesion, the wheal, may be reproduced in approximately 60% of patients by the intradermal injection of autologous serum.[38] Mast cell degranulation has been demonstrated histologically at the site of serum-induced wheals[39] and these sera can release histamine *in vitro* from mast cells derived from human skin[38,40,41] and from other tissues.[41] The serological mediator(s) is also capable of releasing histamine from the basophil leukocytes of healthy donors in 29% of patients.[38] This histamine-releasing activity has been identified as being due to IgG autoantibodies directed either against an epitope or epitopes in the α chain of the high-affinity IgE receptor FcɛRI[30] in 23% of patients,[38] or against IgE in 5.5% of patients.[12,38] Sera from some of the remaining autologous intradermal serum test-positive patients that fail to release histamine from basophil leukocytes have been shown to have a mast cell-specific histamine-releasing activity.[41,42] Although this factor(s) remains to be fully characterized, it can be differentiated from anti-FcɛRIα or anti-IgE antibodies.[41,42]

Of patients with active chronic urticaria 40% have a consistently negative autologous intradermal serum test. Their sera also fail to release histamine *in vitro* from basophil leukocytes[38] and from human skin mast cells.[38,42] The aetiology of the cutaneous whealing in these patients remains unsolved. Thus, at least three pathogenetic subsets of chronic urticaria may be recognized: an autoantibody subset, a mast cell-specific subset, and those with negative skin tests.[37]

## Treatment of chronic urticaria

Antihistamines are the first line of treatment for chronic urticaria, reducing the itching, and the number, size and duration of wheals.[43] The drugs are moderately selective for $H_1$ receptors, blocking them by competitive inhibition.[43] The first-generation $H_1$ receptor antagonists may also antagonize cholinergic, serotoninergic and $\alpha$-adrenergic receptors, but the more specific second-generation antihistamines do not have these effects.[43] However, the response to antihistamine therapy is variable. In a recent survey involving 390 patients attending hospital clinics with chronic urticaria, 44% reported a good response to $H_1$ receptor antagonists.[44]

The therapeutic options for patients with recalcitrant chronic urticaria unresponsive to combinations of antihistamines are limited. Inhibitors of mast cell degranulation, calcium channel blockers, $\beta$-adrenergic stimulants and ultraviolet A irradiation produce inconsistent and frequently disappointing results. A trial of interferon-$\alpha$, which can reduce mast cell proliferation *in vitro*, was also disappointing.[45] The role of corticosteroids in the management of chronic urticaria is debatable.[46] They afford symptomatic relief in the short term, but high doses and prolonged courses of treatment are often necessary.[47] One study has shown that a 7-day course of corticosteroids improves the symptoms of chronic urticaria in association with a decreased production of histamine-releasing factor in blister fluid, although no change was documented for the histamine content of blister fluid on day 7.[48] Many clinicians agree that the use of corticosteroids is limited by their adverse effects[8,9,46,47,49] on hormonal, metabolic and skeletal systems, which occur mainly after prolonged administration.[50] Cyclosporin has been shown to be an effective treatment in a randomized, double-blind study involving 30 chronic urticaria patients with positive autologous intradermal serum tests.[51]

## Intravenous immunoglobulin

Studies of intravenous immunoglobulin (IVIg) in the management of chronic urticaria are summarized (in Table 3.1).[52–54] Our department studied 10 patients with severe, chronic urticaria, which had been present for an average of 33.8 months (range 5–96 months).[52] We aimed to treat a select, homogeneous group. All patients had a positive autologous intradermal serum test and their sera showed positive histamine release from the basophil leukocytes of two healthy donors: the mean (± standard

**Table 3.1**
*Studies of intravenous immunoglobulin (IVIG) in the management of chronic urticaria*

| Reference<br>No. of patients | Treatment<br>regimen | Skin test | Histamine release from<br>donor basophils | Outcome |
|---|---|---|---|---|
| O'Donnell et al, 1998[52]<br>n = 10 | 0.4 g/kg/day<br>× 5 days | Positive<br>n = 10 | Positive<br>n = 10 | Prolonged complete remission, > 3 years (n = 3), temporary remission (n = 2), improvement (n = 4) |
| Asero 2000[53]<br>n = 3 | 0.4 g/kg/day<br>× 5 days | Positive<br>n = 3 | Positive, patient 2<br><br>Negative, patient 1<br>Unknown, patient 3 | Total remission × 3 weeks<br><br>No change<br>Improved control of disease |
| Kroiss et al, 2000[54]<br>n = 1 | 0.2 g/kg<br>× 1 day, repeat at intervals of 4 weeks | Negative<br>n = 1 | | Urticaria suppressed |

deviation) serum-induced histamine release from the basophil leukocytes of donor 1 was 32.4% (± 14.8), and from those of donor 2 was 28.7% (± 16.1). All patients were therefore deemed to have histamine-releasing autoantibodies. Their progress was monitored using an urticaria activity score (range 0–42) based on the number of small and large wheals and the severity of the itch, visual analogue scale and autologous intradermal serum tests. Patients were treated with 0.4 g/kg/day for 5 days.

Patients 1 and 2 showed a striking clinical response, with a complete remission of chronic urticaria which was sustained at the final study visit at 24 weeks posttreatment (Fig. 3.2a) and remains sustained 3 years posttreatment. Three patients (3–5) had a complete remission but relapsed after intervals of 6, 8 (Fig. 3.2b) and 21 weeks, respectively. In patients 6, 7, 8 and 9 their urticaria improved (Fig. 3.2c), and in patient 10 (not illustrated) there was transient improvement only. Patient 5, whose urticaria relapsed after 21 weeks, was retreated and had a prolonged complete remission following a second 5-day course of IVIg (Fig. 3.2d), which is sustained 3 years later. The mean urticaria activity score improved from a baseline value of 24.6 to 12.6 ($P < 0.01$) and 7.8 ($P < 0.01$) at 2 and 6 weeks posttreatment, respectively

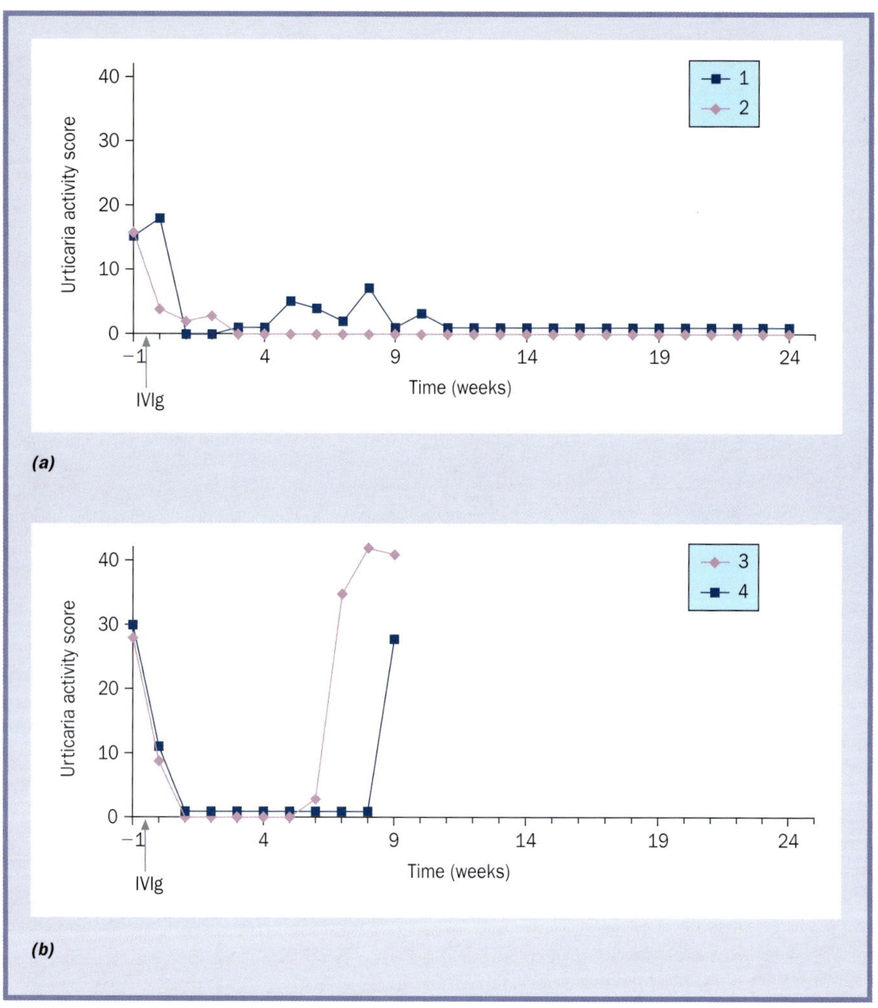


40
30
20
10
0
Urticaria activity score
1
2
−1
4
9
14
19
24
Time (weeks)
IVIg
(a)
40
30
20
10
0
Urticaria activity score
3
4
−1
4
9
14
19
24
Time (weeks)
IVIg
(b)

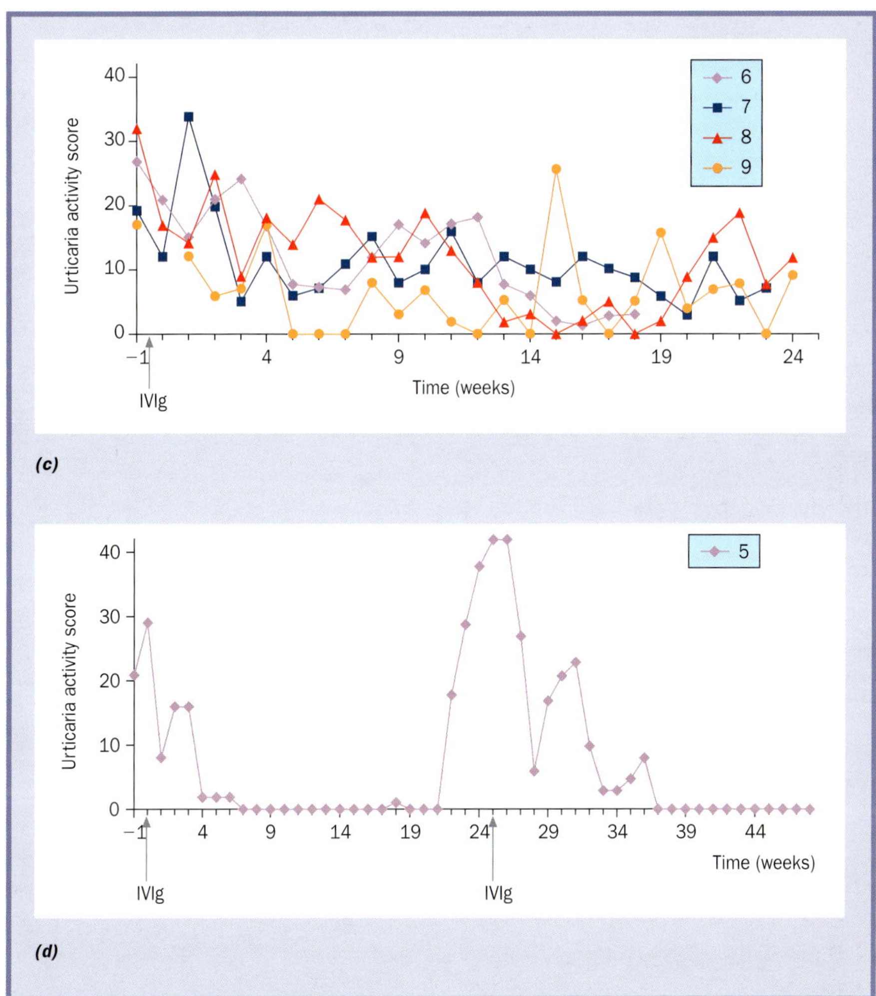


**Fig. 3.2**
*Urticaria activity scores for patients 1 and 2 (a), 3 and 4 (b), and 6, 7, 8, 9 (c) after a single course of IVIg.
(d) The urticaria activity scores for patient 5, who had two courses of IVIg.*

(Wilcoxon's matched pairs). This was mirrored by a significant improvement in the visual analogue scales.

Autologous intradermal serum tests posttreatment showed a reduced or almost absent wheal-and-flare response to post-treatment sera compared to pretreatment sera when the paired sera were tested simultaneously in 7 of 10 patients. Patients who had a complete remission of their urticaria had a negative skin test response to post-treatment serum a number of months post-IVIg (Fig. 3.3). Overall, despite some adverse events and the cost and inconvenience of treatment, we concluded that IVIg represented a therapeutic option in patients with severe autoantibody-mediated chronic urticaria.[52]

Asero[53] treated three patients with skin test-positive chronic urticaria using IVIg 0.4 g/kg/day for 5 days. Interestingly, the single patient (patient 2) who enjoyed total remission of her urticaria for 3 weeks had positive histamine release (9.5%) from donor basophils, and therefore had 'antibody'-type urticaria. Patient 1, whose serum failed to release histamine from donor basophils, had no change in his urticaria. A further patient (patient 3), whose histamine release status was unknown, enjoyed improved control of his disease. Asero concluded that in view of the poor or only temporary clinical effects and expense, 'IVIg cannot be presently regarded as a treatment of choice in patients with severe

chronic idiopathic urticaria'. Kroiss et al.[54] treated one skin test-negative patient with a lower dose of IVIg (0.2 g/kg for 1 day), repeated at intervals of 4 weeks, and noted suppression of the urticaria.

The histamine-releasing activities in the serum of one of our patients before and after IVIg therapy have been studied in detail.[55] The serum-evoked histamine releases from IgE-sensitized and non-sensitized normal human basophils were 31% and 28%, respectively, before IVIg, and 11% and 5%, respectively, 10 weeks posttreatment, when the patient's urticaria was in remission. Preincubation of pre- and post-treatment sera with recombinant soluble human Fc$\epsilon$RI$\alpha$ inhibited histamine release by >35%. Serum-evoked histamine release from human skin slices was 17% before treatment, and declined to 2% at 10 weeks posttreatment. Protein G affinity chromatography of serum demonstrated IgG-dependent and -independent histamine-releasing activities, which declined after IVIg treatment. We concluded that analysis of this patient's serum revealed several biologically active components and that decreases in both total serum histamine-releasing activity and in that due to IgG anti-Fc$\epsilon$RI$\alpha$ autoantibodies were associated with clinical improvement following IVIg therapy.[55]

We studied the effect of IVIg on the course of severe chronic urticaria associated with the novel mast cell-specific histamine-

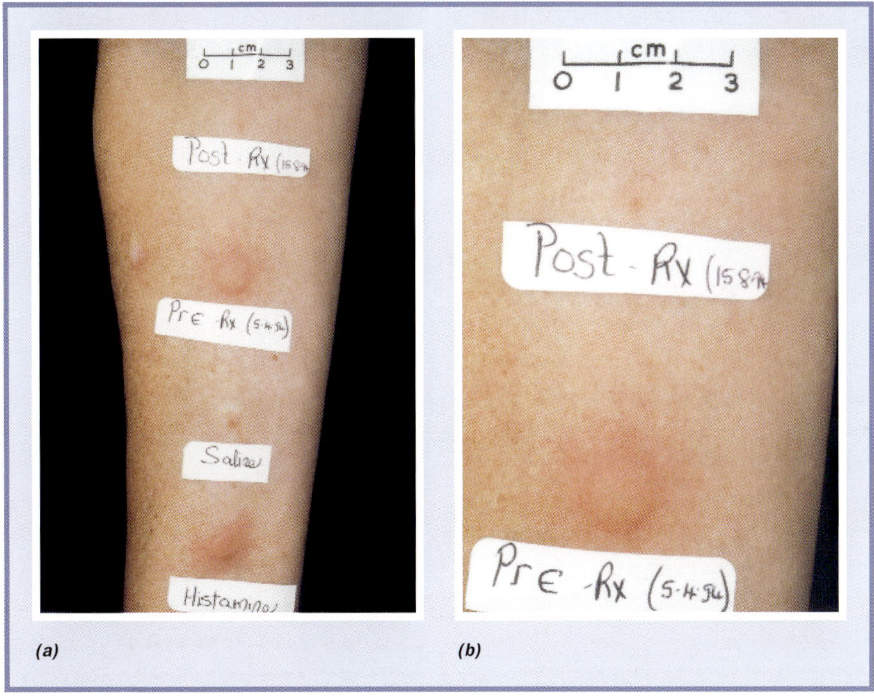



(a)　　　　　(b)

**Fig. 3.3a, b**
*(a) Autologous intradermal serum test posttreatment with IVIg, comparing the response to the intradermal injection of post-treatment serum with the pretreatment serum. The negative (saline) and positive (histamine) controls are also shown. (b) Close-up of cutaneous response to post- and pretreatment serum.*

releasing activity in nine patients (manuscript in preparation). Two patients showed a dramatic response and had a complete remission, which is sustained (> 3 years post-IVIg). Patient 3 had a short, complete remission. Urticarial activity in patients 4–6 diminished, and in patients 7–9 there was transient improvement only.

## Discussion

A single donation of whole blood (400–500 ml) yields approximately 15 ml of plasma proteins, of which only 2–3 ml are Cohn fraction II γ-globulin.[56] The plasma pool from which a batch of IVIg is derived may be obtained from as many as 5000–20,000 donors. The use of different processes to purify immunoglobulin has led to the generation of products similar in immunoglobulin composition but which vary in purity, antibody activity and content of immunomodulatory proteins.[57] Variation in responses to IVIg may reflect 'lot to lot' variation in the product, differences in disease pathogenesis or subset, or other individual disease factors, for example the non-specific aggravation of chronic urticaria by stress, hormonal factors, diet and drugs. In treating chronic urticaria we used the dosage recommended by the manufacturer for the treatment of idiopathic thrombocytopenic purpura. However, the optimum dose of IVIg has not been determined for a number of its established indications.[58]

The subset of chronic urticaria patients whose disease is caused by histamine-releasing autoantibodies may benefit from manipulation of the immune system. Plasmapheresis offers temporary response in some patients, but is unlikely to prevent the reaccumulation of the autoantibodies.[59] IVIg is a less expensive and less invasive option, and our study indicates that it offers the possibility of a prolonged remission in patients with otherwise treatment-resistant chronic urticaria.[52] IVIg differs significantly from other immunosuppressive agents and represents a novel therapy for the dysfunctional immune system in a number of autoimmune diseases. In idiopathic thrombocytopenic purpura blockade of

receptors for the Fc portion of IgG molecules on reticuloendothelial cells, inhibiting the destruction of autoantibody-coated platelets, has been demonstrated after treatment with IVIg.[60] Others, using peripheral blood mononuclear cells, suggested that blockade of the reticuloendothelial system by IVIg was the result of a decrease in Fc receptor affinity and a competitive interaction between the increasing levels of serum IgG from the infusion of IVIg and IgG-coated platelets, for the Fc receptor.[61] In anti-factor VIIIc autoimmune disease, treatment with IVIg resulted in a dramatic and prolonged suppression of antibody, which was also demonstrated *in vitro.*[62] The recovery of patients post-IVIg was ascribed to the generation of antiidiotypes against anti-factor VIIIc antibodies.[62] A neutralizing activity against anti-factor VIII autoantibodies was detected in pools of IgG of as few as two to four donors, of whom individually tested IgG did not exhibit inhibitory activity against anti-factor VIII autoantibodies.[63] IVIg is known to induce a fall in autoantibody titres, for example anti-DNA,[64,65] antithyroglobulin,[65] anti-intrinsic factor[65] and ANCA.[66] The presence of anti-idiotypic antibodies to ANCA in IVIg and in remission sera from patients with systemic vasculitis suggests a role for idiotypic regulation in the normal control of these disorders.[66] In chronic urticaria mediated by functionally significant autoantibodies, IVIg may provide anti-idiotypic antibodies capable of suppressing histamine-releasing autoantibodies. A direct inhibitory effect on B-cell function and/or T-cell function may also explain some of the response.[67] It has also been suggested that IVIg may accelerate the degradation of IgG, thereby reducing the levels of pathogenic autoantibodies.[68]

The mechanism of IVIg in the subset of patients with chronic urticaria in association with a mast cell-specific histamine-releasing activity is speculative, and although six of the nine patients' urticaria improved, the beneficial effects were less clear-cut than in patients with autoimmune chronic urticaria.

Adverse effects to IVIg have been ascribed to the presence of residual impurities (acid proteinases, kinins and isohaemagglutinins), aggregated immunoglobulin molecules, antigen–antibody reactions, or to possible contaminants or stabilizers that may have been used during the manufacturing process.[69] The incidence of adverse events is reported by the manufacturers to be in the range of 1–15% (usually less than 5%),[70] but may be higher in hypogammaglobulinaemic patients.[71] The reactions are reportedly mild and self-limited.[70] In our experience adverse effects of IVIg were more frequent and severe than anticipated, and usually developed on days 2 or 3. Headache was the commonest complaint, and in two patients had features of aseptic meningitis, a recognized complication of IVIg, more common in those with a past history of migraine.[72] One patient developed classic symptoms of migraine, which has also previously been reported.[73] Nausea, low-grade pyrexia, phlebitis at the intravenous infusion site, flu-like symptoms and lethargy also occurred. In addition, two patients showed transient elevation of liver enzymes. Transient increases in alanine transferase and other liver enzymes, not associated with hepatitis A, B or C, are a recognized finding post-IVIg,[74,75] but are of uncertain significance (Sandoz, personal communication).

Of our patients treated with IVIg, five developed vesicular hand eczema. Histological examination of a punch biopsy skin sample was consistent with an eczematous reaction. The rash, which commenced on days 3–5 of the IVIg infusions, responded to moderately potent topical steroids. Three reports of 'pompholyx eczema' have been received by the manufacturers of *Sandoglobulin* (Sandoz, personal communication, 1994), and a generalized eczematous reaction has been noted following repeat infusions of IVIg.[76] The manufacturers of *Alphaglobin* received no reports of eczema (Alpha, personal communication, 1996).

The frequency of side-effects in the urticaria population may make a double-blind evaluation of the role of IVIg in the management of chronic urticaria difficult. However, the therapeutic options for severe chronic urticaria which is unresponsive to antihistamines are limited. Preliminary experience with IVIg is promising. The studies underlie the importance of studying subsets of chronic urticaria with different types of histamine-releasing activity separately. Placebo-controlled trials are warranted in patients with autoimmune chronic urticaria, and ideally would also be carried out in patients with the mast cell-specific histamine-releasing activity. IVIg represents an important therapeutic option in patients with severe, treatment-resistant, antibody-positive chronic urticaria.

## Acknowledgement

IVIg studies[52,55] were carried out at the Professional Unit, St John's Institute of Dermatology, St Thomas' Hospital, London. I am very grateful to Professor Malcolm W Greaves for his support.

## References

1. Champion RH, Pye RJ. Urticaria – clinical aspects. In: Champion RH, Greaves MW, Kobza Black A, Pye RJ, eds. *The Urticarias.* London: Churchill Livingstone, 1985: 135–40.

2. Champion RH, Roberts SOB, Carpenter RG et al. Urticaria and angio-oedema. A review of 554 patients. *Br J Dermatol* 1969; **81:** 588–97.

3. Green GR, Koelsche GA, Kierland RR. Etiology and pathogenesis of chronic urticaria. *Ann Allergy* 1965; **23:** 30–6.

4. Greaves MW, O'Donnell BF. Not all chronic urticaria is 'idiopathic'! *Exp Dermatol* 1998; **7:** 11–13.

5. Hide M, Francis DM, Grattan CEH et al. The pathogenesis of chronic idiopathic urticaria: new evidence suggests an auto-immune basis and implications for treatment. *Clin Exp Allergy* 1994; **24:** 624–7.

6. Grattan CEH, Francis DM. Autoimmune urticaria. *Adv Dermatol* 1999; **15:** 311–40.

7. Grattan CEH, Sabroe RA, Greaves MW. Chronic urticaria. *J Am Acad Dermatol* 2002; **46:** 645–57.

8. Monroe EW. Urticaria. *Curr Probl Dermatol* 1993; **5:** 118–40.

9. Greaves MW. Chronic urticaria. *N Engl J Med* 1995; **332:** 1767–72.

10. Czarnetzki BM. Acute and chronic urticaria. In: Czarnetzki BM, ed. *Urticaria.* Berlin: Springer-Verlag, 1986: 26–46.

11. Sabroe RA, Seed PT, Francis DM et al. Chronic idiopathic urticaria: comparison of the clinical features of patients with and without anti-FcεRI or anti-IgE autoantibodies. *J Am Acad Dermatol* 1999; **40:** 443–50.

12. Grattan CEH, Francis DM, Hide M et al. Detection of circulating histamine releasing autoantibodies with functional properties of anti-IgE in chronic urticaria. *Clin Exp Allergy* 1991; **21:** 695–704.

13. O'Donnell BF, Lawlor F, Simpson J et al. The impact of chronic urticaria on the quality of life. *Br J Dermatol* 1997; **136:** 197–201.

14. Dolovich J, Hargreave FE, Chalmers R et al. Late cutaneous allergic responses in isolated IgE-dependent reactions. *J Allergy Clin Immunol* 1973; **52:** 38–46.

15. Solley GO, Gleich GJ, Jordan RE et al. The late phase of the immediate wheal and flare skin reaction: its dependence upon IgE antibodies. *J Clin Invest* 1976; **58**: 408–20.

16. Mathews KP. Chronic urticaria. In: Schocket AL ed. *Clinical Management of Urticaria and Anaphylaxis.* New York: Marcel Dekker, 1993: 21–68.

17. Czarnetzki BM. Basic mechanisms. In: Czarnetzki BM, ed. *Urticaria.* Berlin: Springer-Verlag, 1986: 5–25.

18. Rothe MJ, Nowak M, Kerdel FA. The mast cell in health and disease. *J Am Acad Dermatol* 1990; **23**: 615–24.

19. Schwartz LB. Mast cells and their role in urticaria. *J Am Acad Dermatol* 1991; **25**: 190–204.

20. Natbony SF, Phillips ME, Elias JM et al. Histologic studies of chronic idiopathic urticaria. *J Allergy Clin Immunol* 1983; **71**: 177–83.

21. Smith CH, Kepley C, Schwartz LB et al. Mast cell number and phenotype in chronic idiopathic urticaria. *J Allergy Clin Immunol* 1995; **96**: 360–4.

22. Kaplan AP, Horakova Z, Katz SI. Assessment of tissue fluid histamine levels in patients with urticaria. *J Allergy Clin Immunol* 1978; **61**: 350–4.

23. Phanuphak P, Schocket AL, Arroyave CM et al. Skin histamine in chronic urticaria. *J Allergy Clin Immunol* 1980; **65**: 371–5.

24. Maxwell DL, Atkinson BA, Spur BW et al. Skin responses to intradermal histamine and leukotrienes $C_4$, $D_4$, and $E_4$ in patients with chronic idiopathic urticaria and in normal subjects. *J Allergy Clin Immunol* 1990; **86**: 759–65.

25. Bressler RB. Pathophysiology of chronic urticaria. *Immunol Allergy Clin North Am* 1995; **15**: 659–77.

26. Claveau J, Lavoie A, Brunet C et al. Chronic idiopathic urticaria: possible contribution of histamine-releasing factor to pathogenesis. *J Allergy Clin Immunol* 1993; **92**: 132–7.

27. Nitschke M, Sohn K, Dieckmann D et al. Effects of basophil-priming and stimulating cytokines on histamine release from isolated human skin mast cells. *Arch Dermatol Res* 1996; **288**: 463–8.

28. Grattan CEH, Wallington TB, Warin RP et al. A serological mediator in chronic idiopathic urticaria – a clinical, immunological and histological evaluation. *Br J Dermatol* 1986; **114**: 583–90.

29. Grattan CEH, Hamon CGB, Cowan MA et al. Preliminary identification of a low molecular weight serological mediator in chronic idiopathic urticaria. *Br J Dermatol* 1988; **119**: 179–84.

30. Hide M, Francis DM, Grattan CEH et al. Autoantibodies against the high-affinity IgE receptor as a cause of histamine release in chronic urticaria. *N Engl J Med* 1993; **328**: 1599–604.

31. Greaves MW, O'Donnell BF, Winkelmann RK. Chronic urticaria – evidence for autoimmunity. *Allergy Clin Immunol News* 1995; **7**: 36–8.

32. Fiebiger E, Maurer D, Holub H et al. Serum IgG autoantibodies directed against the α chain of FcεRI: a selective marker and pathogenetic factor for a distinct subset of chronic urticaria patients? *J Clin Invest* 1995; **96**: 2606–12.

33. Rorsman H. Basophilic leucopenia in different forms of urticaria. *Acta Allergol* 1962; **17**: 168–84.

34. Witebsky E, Rose NR, Terplan K et al. Chronic thyroiditis and autoimmunization. *JAMA* 1957; **164**: 1439–47.

35. Rose NR, Bona C. Defining criteria for autoimmune diseases (Witebsky's postulates revisited). *Immunol Today* 1993; **14**: 426–30.

36. Rose NR. Foreword - The uses of autoantibodies. In: Peter JB, Shoenfeld Y, eds. *Autoantibodies.* Amsterdam: Elsevier 1996; xxvii–xxix.

37. O'Donnell BF, O'Neill CM, Francis DM et al. Human leucocyte antigen class II associations in chronic idiopathic urticaria. *Br J Dermatol* 1999; **140**: 853–8

38. Niimi N, Francis DM, Kermani F et al. Dermal mast activation by autoantibodies against the high affinity IgE receptor in chronic urticaria. *J Invest Dermatol* 1996; **106**: 1001–6.

39. Grattan CEH, Boon AP, Eady RAJ et al. The pathology of the autologous serum skin test response in chronic urticaria resembles IgE-mediated late-phase reactions. *Int Arch Allergy Appl Immunol* 1990; **93**: 198–204.

40. Francis DM, Niimi N, Hide M et al. Histamine release from human skin *in vitro* induced by sera containing IgG anti-FcɛRIα autoantibodies from patients with chronic urticaria. *J Invest Dermatol* 1994; **103**: 399 [abst].

41. Kermani F, Niimi N, Francis DM et al. Characterization of a novel mast cell-specific histamine releasing activity in chronic idiopathic urticaria (CIU). *J Invest Dermatol* 1995; **105**: 452 [abst].

42. Niimi N, Kermani F, Francis DM et al. Mast cell specific histamine releasing activity in chronic idiopathic urticaria (CIU). *J Invest Dermatol* 1995; **104**: 572 [abst].

43. Simons FER, Simons KJ. The pharmacology and use of H₁-receptor-antagonist drugs. *N Engl J Med* 1994; **330**: 1663–70.

44. Humphreys F, Hunter JAA. The characteristics of urticaria in 390 patients. *Br J Dermatol* 1998; **138**: 635–8.

45. Czarnetzki BM, Algermissen B, Jeep S et al. Interferon treatment of patients with chronic urticaria and mastocytosis. *J Am Acad Dermatol* 1994; **30**: 500–1.

46. Warin RP, Champion RH. Acute and chronic urticaria: treatment. In: Warin RP, Champion RH, eds. *Urticaria.* London: WB Saunders, 1974: 100–12.

47. Thompson JS. Urticaria and angioedema. *Ann Intern Med* 1968; **69**: 361–80.

48. Paradis L, Lavoie A, Brunet C et al. Effects of systemic corticosteroids on cutaneous histamine secretion and histamine-releasing factor in patients with chronic idiopathic urticaria. *Clin Exp Allergy* 1996; **26**: 815–20.

49. Kennard CD, Ellis CN. Pharmacologic therapy for urticaria. *J Am Acad Dermatol* 1991; **25**: 176–89.

50. Siegel SC. Overview of corticosteroid therapy. *J Allergy Clin Immunol* 1985; **76**: 312–20.

51. Grattan CEH, O'Donnell BF, Francis DM et al. Randomized double-blind study of cyclosporin in chronic 'idiopathic' urticaria. *Br J Dermatol* 2000; **143**: 365–72.

52. O'Donnell BF, Barr RM, Kobza Black A et al. Intravenous immunoglobulin (IVIG) in autoimmune chronic urticaria. *Br J Dermatol* 1998; **138**: 101–6.

53. Asero R. Are IVIG for chronic unremitting urticaria effective? *Allergy* 2000; **55**: 1099–101.

54. Kroiss M, Vogt T, Landthaler M et al. The

effectiveness of low-dose intravenous immunoglobulin in chronic urticaria. *Acta Dermatol Venereol* 2000; **80**: 225 [letter].

55. Niimi N, Kermani F, Francis DM et al. Serum anti-FcεRI histamine releasing activity in chronic urticaria treated by intravenous immunoglobulin. *J Invest Dermatol* 1994; **103**: 400 [abst].

56. Greenbaum BH. Differences in immunoglobulin preparations for intravenous use: a comparison of six products. *Am J Pediatr Hematol Oncol* 1990; **12**: 490–6.

57. Lam L, Whitsett CF, McNicholl JM et al. Immunologically active proteins in intravenous immunoglobulin. *Lancet* 1993; **342**: 678.

58. Bussel JB, Fitzgerald-Pedersen J, Feldman C. Alternation of two doses of intravenous gammaglobulin in the maintenance treatment of patients with immune thrombocytopenic purpura: more is not always better. *Am J Hematol* 1990; **33**: 184–8.

59. Grattan CEH, Francis DM, Slater NGP et al. Plasmapheresis for severe, unremitting, chronic urticaria. *Lancet* 1992; **339**: 1078–80.

60. Clarkson SB, Bussel JB, Kimberly RP et al. Treatment of refractory immune thrombocytopenic purpura with an anti-Fcγ-receptor antibody. *N Engl J Med* 1986; **314**: 1236–9.

61. Kimberly RP, Salmon JE, Bussel JB et al. Modulation of mononuclear phagocyte functions by intravenous γ-globulin. *J Immunol* 1984; **132**: 745–50.

62. Sultan Y, Kazatchkine MD, Maisonneuve P et al. Anti-idiotypic suppression of autoantibodies to factor VIII (antihaemophilic factor) by high-dose intravenous gammaglobulin. *Lancet* 1984; **ii**: 765–8.

63. Dietrich G, Algiman M, Sultan Y et al. Origin of anti-idiotypic activity against anti-factor VIII autoantibodies in pools of normal human immunoglobulin (IVIg). *Blood* 1992; **79**: 2946–51.

64. Abdou NI, Wall H, Lindsley HB et al. Network theory in autoimmunity. In vitro suppression of serum anti-DNA antibody binding to DNA by anti-idiotypic antibody in systemic lupus erythematosus. *J Clin Invest* 1981; **67**: 1297–304.

65. Rossi F, Kazatchkine MD. Antiidiotypes against autoantibodies in pooled normal human polyspecific Ig. *J Immunol* 1989; **143**: 4104–9.

66. Jayne DRW, Esnault VLM, Lockwood CM. ANCA anti-idiotype antibodies and the treatment of systemic vasculitis with intravenous immunoglobulin. *J Autoimmunity* 1993; **6**: 207–19.

67. Dwyer JM. Manipulating the immune system with immune globulin. *N Engl J Med* 1992; **326**: 107–16.

68. Yu Z, Lennon VA. Mechanism of intravenous immune globulin therapy in antibody-mediated autoimmune diseases. *N Engl J Med* 1999; **340**: 227–8.

69. Duhem C, Dicato MA, Ries F. Side-effects of intravenous immune globulins. *Clin Exp Immunol* 1994; **97** (Suppl 1): 79–83.

70. NIH Consensus Conference. Intravenous immunoglobulin. Prevention and treatment of disease. *JAMA* 1990; **264**: 3189–93.

71. Lederman HM, Roifman CM, Lavi S et al. Corticosteroids for prevention of adverse reactions to intravenous immune serum globulin infusions in hypogammaglobulinemic patients. *Am J Med* 1986; **81**: 443–6.

72. Sekul EA, Cupler EJ, Dalakas MC. Aseptic meningitis associated with high-dose intravenous immunoglobulin therapy: frequency and risk factors. *Ann Intern Med* 1994; **121**: 259–62.

73. Constantinescu CS, Chang AP, McCluskey LF. Recurrent migraine and intravenous immune globulin therapy. *N Engl J Med* 1993; **329**: 583–4.

74. Hany M, Ryan A, Webster ADB. Long-term safety and tolerability of intravenous immunoglobulin. *Lancet* 1991; **338**: 194–5.

75. Zuhrie SR, Webster ADB, Davies R et al. A prospective controlled crossover trial of a new heat-treated intravenous immunoglobulin. *Clin Exp Immunol* 1995; **99**: 10–15.

76. Barucha C, McMillan JC. Eczema after intravenous infusion of immunoglobulin. *Br Med J* 1987; **295**: 1141 (letter).

# Atopic dermatitis – role of hdIVIg

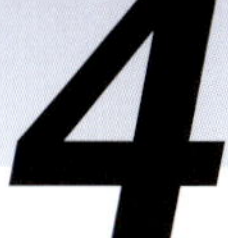

## Samantha Eisman and Malcolm HA Rustin

AD, atopic dermatitis; ECP, eosinophil cationic protein; ELAM, endothelial leukocyte adhesion molecule; hdIVIg, high-dose intravenous immunoglobulin; ICAM, intercellular adhesion molecule; ITP, idiopathic thrombocytopenic purpura

## Introduction

Atopic dermatitis (AD) is one of the commonest skin diseases, affecting 20% of children and, with its chronic relapsing nature, about 6% of adults (Fig. 4.1). Treatment generally relies on a balance between control of the condition, quality of life and safe long-term treatment. Successful treatment can usually be obtained in mild to moderate disease with topical preparations, by decreasing trigger factors and by management of allergies (Fig. 4.2). For recalcitrant cases, systemic therapies are available but are limited by their toxicity and efficacy. It is for these patients that therapeutic advances are sought. High-dose intravenous immunoglobulin (hdIVIg) has been noted to be beneficial in the treatment of AD anecdotally, in case

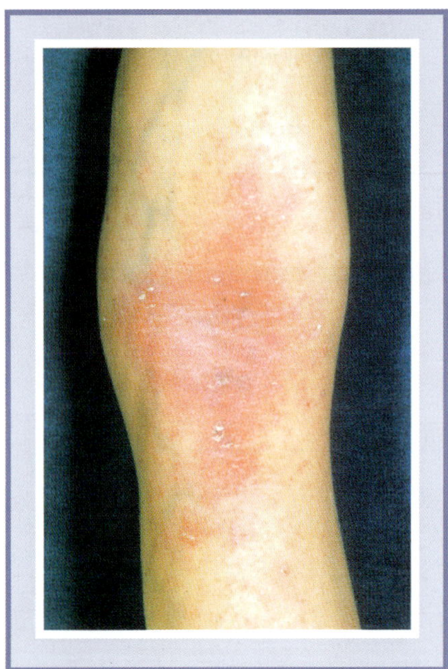

**Fig. 4.1**
*Typical flexural involvement in atopic dermatitis.*

reports and in small uncontrolled trials. As yet, no double-blind placebo-controlled studies have been performed.

## Evidence in the literature

Kimata[1] first described the benefits of hdIVIg when an incidental improvement in severe AD was noted in four children treated with hdIVIg (0.4 g/kg/day for 5 days) as sole therapy for Kawasaki disease and idiopathic thrombocytopenic purpura (ITP). All four experienced at least a 50% improvement in their AD by day 7, and near complete remission by day 14. Improvement was noted in skin scores and sleep patterns, and a decrease in IgE level, *in vitro* spontaneous IgE production and eosinophil counts were recorded. At 6 months the two patients with Kawasaki disease had no further treatment

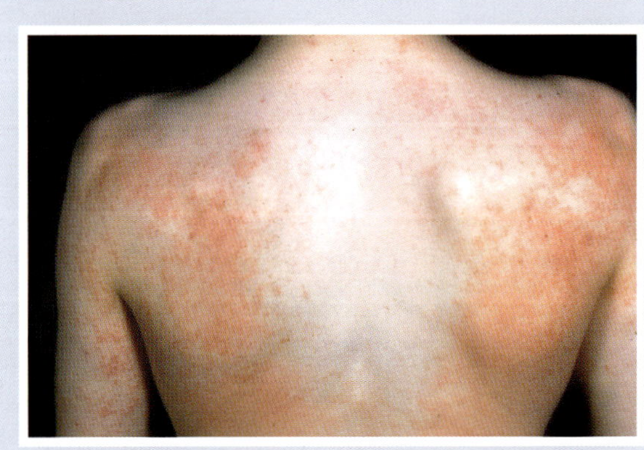

**Fig. 4.2**
*Generalized untreated atopic dermatitis.*

requirements for their AD, and similarly at 1 year the two patients with ITP were no longer reliant on treatment.

An open trial assessing the benefits of hdIVIg in allergic patients was performed by Gelfand et al.[2] Three patients with severe AD despite oral and highly potent topical steroids, were treated with hdIVIg 2 g/kg/month for 6 months. Improvement in symptom scores was mirrored by clinical clearance in serial photographs. A rapid reduction in pruritus was noted, serum IgE levels were unchanged. Interestingly, cessation of the hdIVIg at 6 months was associated with a recurrence of symptoms, which disappeared on reinstitution of the treatment. Reduction in concurrent steroid treatment was not described.

A report by Weiss et al.[3] revealed no improvement in the AD of an 8-month-old boy treated with a single cycle of hdIVIg, 1 g/kg, for Wiskott–Aldrich syndrome, a primary immunodeficiency syndrome.

Another open study by Wakim et al.[4] treated nine patients with AD and one with hyper-IgE syndrome with hdIVIg, 2 g/kg/month for 7 months. One patient was withdrawn from the study because of a serum sickness-type reaction. The remaining patients tolerated the infusions, but no statistical improvement in skin scores was demonstrated. In fact, skin scores improved slightly in six patients, were unchanged in two and worsened in one. There was a non-

significant reduction in serum IgE levels, and allergen-specific IgE levels were unaltered.

A larger study was conducted by Noh and Lee[5] recruiting 41 patients with severe steroid-resistant AD who were given a single cycle of low-dose IVIg. Patients received 0.5 g/kg if they weighed less than 30 kg and 15 g if they weighed more than 30kg. There was a pretreatment washout period in which no topical or systemic steroids were allowed and systemic therapy was prohibited. Disease severity was significantly decreased by day 7, and was still significantly lower at day 14 compared to day 0 levels. There was an associated reduction in serum IgE levels. Unfortunately, these patients had a short and variable follow-up period and therefore long-term benefits were not documented. In addition, these authors used low doses of IVIg.

Jolles et al.[6] analysed the cytokines in stimulated and unstimulated cells in an AD patient to determine a possible mechanism of action of IVIg. One patient with severe AD taking prednisolone and hydroxychloroquine received adjunctive hdIVIg 0.4 g/kg/day for 5 days, and over a 10-month period the monthly infusions were given over 2 days. An initial increase in IL-4-positive cells on day 4 of a 5-day treatment course was observed, mirrored by a similar peak in the unstimulated cells. No significant change in IL-2 or IFN-$\gamma$-positive CD4 T cells was noted. IL-4 production was found to decline over the following 2 weeks and the patient's skin score declined over this period despite a severe episode of eczema herpeticum and staphylococcal infection. A gradual fall in specific IgE radioallergosorbent test to house dust mite and cat dander was also observed.

Jolles et al.[7] treated three patients suffering from severe AD with hdIVIg 2 g/kg/month for 11 months. All had steroid-induced osteoporosis, but were allowed to continue on the same dose of prednisolone or combined prednisolone and hydroxychloroquine. All experienced a significant reduction in skin scores, but IgE level declined in only one patient. All three patients managed to taper or stop their oral prednisolone requirements.

Huang et al.[8] evaluated the effect of intravenous immunoglobulin (2 g/kg/month) in five children aged 7–12 months with severe intractable AD, most of whom had required systemic steroids for control of their skin disease. Three cycles were administered and patients were allowed to continue topical steroid treatment. A marked and consistent improvement of clinical symptoms was noted in all children, and discontinuation of treatment did not result in relapse in any of them. Decreased levels of intercellular adhesion molecule 1 (ICAM-1), endothelial leukocyte adhesion molecule 1 (ELAM-1) and eosinophil cationic protein (ECP) were noted in patients receiving hdIVIg, compared to AD controls not treated with IVIg and normal controls. No significant difference was

detected in CD4$^+$ T-cell intracellular IFN-$\gamma$ or IL-4 levels.

In a further study,[9] six patients with AD were treated with adjunctive hdIVIg 2 g/kg/month for 6 months, meaning that all patients continued with second-line agents (azathioprine, prednisolone or hydroxychloroquine). Four out of the six patients had significant improvement in their skin scores. Lymphocyte phenotypes showed a decrease in CD4 T cells following the immunoglobulin infusions, which had recovered by the next cycle. CD69 expression in both CD4$^+$ and CD8$^+$ cells decreased during the 6 months of hdIVIg therapy to 60% of baseline values, but this was not of statistical significance. The proinflammatory cytokines IFN-$\gamma$ and TNF-$\alpha$ were studied in the CD4 and CD8 populations and no significant changes were noted.

Paul et al[10] recently performed a randomized evaluator-blinded trial in 10 patients with severe AD. After stopping immunosuppressive treatment, oral corticosteroids or phototherapy, 1 month prior to starting the study, patients received either immediate or delayed (1 month) treatment with hdIVIg 2 g/kg. This was administered as an 8 hour infusion over 2 days. At day 30 after infusion, no significant difference in the severity scoring of AD was noted (SCORAD), however a statistically significant improvement of 22% in the SCORAD index was noted at 60 days in the cohort as a whole. No clinically significant change in global evaluation of disease severity by patients was documented and no change in serum IgE levels was observed. It was concluded that one course of hdIVIg given as monotherapy did not modify the clinical course of severe AD in adults in this small study.

## Summary

In total, there are only 42 patients in the literature who have been treated with hdIVIg, 17 of whom had concomitant adjunctive therapy (Table 4.1). The data obtained in most of these few case reports and uncontrolled studies represent small numbers, and this should be borne in mind when conclusions are drawn. There is likely to be reporting bias for successful outcomes, inequalities between study scoring systems of AD, as well as measures of AD severity at the time of treatment.

Jolles[11] looked separately at the response of adults versus children with AD who received hdIVIg. In the above reports, 10 children, under 6 years of age have received hdIVIg as monotherapy: 90% of children responded to treatment with benefits lasting 6 months. The longest response time was noted to be 3 months. An ideal trial for children would therefore be a double-blind placebo-controlled trial employing hdIVIg as monotherapy and lasting more than 3 months before efficacy is assessed, and parameters measured should include photographic documentation, skin scores and laboratory indices that would appear to correlate with improvement after treatment, namely a decrease in eosinophil counts, ECP, IgE, ICAM-1 and ELAM-1.

Fourteen adults were treated with monotherapy and none were shown to have significant disease improvement. Seventeen received adjunctive treatment. Ten of these 17 were noted to have a significant improvement, with responses occurring between 2 and 4 months after the initiation of treatment, but long-lasting remission was observed in a minority of cases only. Five patients with no significant improvement were on less than 7 mg of adjunctive prednisolone a day, a dose unlikely to be synergistic with IVIg or to be capable of disease control in resistant cases. From the above reports it is difficult to ascertain which adult cases would be likely to benefit from treatment, or which markers of disease activity should be utilized. Recently Paul et al[10] performed the first randomized study using hdIVIg in AD. In this study hdIVIg was given as a single dose of monotherapy, however in dermatological conditions, including AD, IVIg has been shown to be more effective when used as adjunctive therapy. The study was of a small size and also of short duration. The half-life of IgG is 11–17 days and it may take 2–4 months to establish evidence of benefit for dermatological conditions, including AD. In view of this and despite this being a randomized study, it is not possible to draw

**Table 4.1**
hdIVIg in atopic dermatitis.

| Number of patients | Demographics | Dose & frequency | IVIg preparation | Additional treatment | Outcome | Response time | Duration of remission | Reference |
|---|---|---|---|---|---|---|---|---|
| 2M, 2F | 2–6 yrs | 0.4 g/kg for 5 days | N/A | Monotherapy | All improved | 4–7 days | 6 months | 1 |
| 3M, 2F | 7–12 months | 2 g/kg/month for 3 cycles | Bayer Biological Co. | Monotherapy | All improved | 3 months | > 6 months | 6 |
| 1M (WAS) | 8 months | 1 g/kg for 1 cycle | N/A | Monotherapy | No improvement | N/A | N/A | 3 |
| 6M | 18–53 yrs | 2 g/kg/month for 6 cycles | Flebogamma® | Adjunctive, Aza, Pred or Hxc | 4 of 6 improved | 2–4 months | 2 of 4 more than 3/12 | 9 |
| 10 patients (1 with HIGE) | 7–64 yrs | 2 g/kg/month for 7 cycles | Venoglobulin-I® | Pred <7 mg/d in 5 Monotherapy in 4 (9 completed study) | Non-significant improvement in 6/9 (2 unchanged, worse in 1) | N/A | N/A | 4 |
| 3M | 19–45 yrs | 2 g/kg/month for 11 cycles | Sandoglobulin® & Alphaglobin® | Adjunctive, Pred, Hxc | All improved | 2–4 months with maximal benefit at 11 months | 1 longlasting and 2 having IVIg 8 weekly | 7 |
| 3 patients | 31–40 yrs | 2 g/kg/month for 6 cycles | N/A | Pred | All improved | N/A | Shortlived | 2 |
| 6M, 4F | 21–38 yrs | 1 g/kg/day for 2 consecutive days only | Sandoglobulin® | Monotherapy | No significant improvement | N/A | N/A | 10 |

WAS: Wiskott Aldrich Syndrome, HIGE: Hyper IgE syndrome, Pred: prednisolone, Aza: Azashiaprime, Hxc: Hydroxycloroquine, N/A: not available conclusions for or against hdIVIg in refractory AD from this data. A large double-blind placebo-controlled trial of hdIVIg and adjunctive treatment should therefore be carried out in adults with AD to assess the role of hdIVIg in the management of recalcitrant patients.

## Discussion

Th2-type cells play a key role in AD.[12] In early, acute AD it has been proposed that a Th2 profile is dominant and that IVIg may modulate cytokines and cytokine antagonists and direct a Th2-mediated disease towards a Th1 cytokine profile, dominant in chronic AD. Jolles et al.[6] demonstrated a decrease in IL-4, a Th2 cytokine, following HdIVIg, which may explain how IVIg acts in the acute phase of AD. Huang et al.[8] did not find that IVIg therapy influenced the balance of Th1/Th2 in AD patients. This may be due to the fact that in their study, patients had a decreased percentage of Th2 cells and a higher Th1/Th2 ratio to start with compared with healthy controls, suggesting that their patients had more chronic lesions at the start of the trial. In addition, analysis of cytokine expression profiles from blood-derived lymphocytes may not reflect changes occurring in T cells infiltrating the skin.

Another possible mechanism of action is the antibacterial and antitoxin effects of IVIg against superantigens produced by staphylococci, which may be contributing to inflammation in AD. Neutralizing these toxins may reduce the capacity to trigger the large number of T cells to release cytokines causing inflammation. IVIg may also reduce the influx of inflammatory cells into the skin in active dermatitis, as is evident by a decrease in levels of ICAM-1, ELAM-1 and ECP, correlating with an improvement in disease.[8]

Bjork et al.[13] showed downregulation of IFN-$\gamma$ production by IVIg, in contrast to the studies cited above. Thepen et al.[14] noted that IFN-$\gamma$ mRNA and protein were highly expressed in 80% of eczematous skin in AD patients. Increased IFN-$\gamma$ has been reported in chronic AD lesions, determining the severity of disease.[15] This may be yet a further mechanism of action of IVIg.

IVIg contains anti-Fas antibodies, which appear to block Fas interactions. T cell-mediated Fas-induced keratinocyte apoptosis has recently been described in AD,[16] and may also be important in the mode of operation of IVIg.

Other possible mechanisms of action include alterations in the recirculation of skin homing T cells, alteration in co-stimulatory molecules (CD28/CD40) required for proliferation, and modulation of IgE-mediated responses and a reduction of IgE synthesis.[17]

There are many theories as to how IVIg works, but further research is required to understand this complex field better. hdIVIg offers an attractive therapeutic option because of its excellent safety record, and it avoids the side effects of steroids and other immunosuppressive agents. Further potential advances in the treatment of AD with hdIVIg will require careful patient selection and appropriately designed placebo-controlled randomized studies.

## References


1.  Kimata H. High dose gammaglobulin treatment for atopic dermatitis. *Arch Dis Child* 1994; **70**: 335–6.

2.  Gelfand EW, Landwehr LP, Esterl B, Mazer B. Intravenous immune globulin: an alternative therapy in steroid-dependent allergic diseases. *Clin Exp Immunol* 1996; **104**: (Suppl 1) 61–6.

3.  Weiss SJ, Schuval SJ, Bonagura VR. Eczema and thrombocytopenia in an 8–month-old infant boy. *Ann Allergy Asthma Immunol* 1997; **78**: 179–82.

4.  Wakim M, Alazard M, Yajima A, Speights D, Saxon A, Stiehm AR. High dose intravenous immunoglobulin in atopic dermatitis and hyper-IgE syndrome. *Ann Allergy Asthma Immunol* 1998; **81**: 153–8.

5.  Noh G, Lee KY. Intravenous immune globulin (IVIG) therapy in steroid-resistant atopic dermatitis. *J Korean Med Sci* 1996; **14**: 63–8.

6.  Jolles S, Hughes J, Rustin M. Intracellular interleukin-4 profiles during high-dose intravenous immunoglobulin treatment of therapy-resistant atopic dermatitis. *J Am Acad Dermatol* 1999; **40**:121–3.

7.  Jolles S, Hughes J, Rustin M. The treatment of atopic dermatitis with adjunctive high-dose intravenous immunoglobulin: a report of three patients and review of the literature. *Br J Dermatol* 2000; **142**: 551–4.

8.  Huang J, Lee W, Chen L, Kuo M, Hsieh K. Changes of serum levels of interleukin-2, intercellular adhesion molecule-1, endothelial leukocyte adhesion molecule-1 and Th1 and Th2 cell in severe atopic dermatitis after intravenous immunoglobulin therapy. *Ann Allergy Asthma Immunol* 2000; **84**: 345–52.

9.  Jolles S, Sewell C, Webster D et al. Adjunctive high-dose intravenous immunoglobulin (HdIVIg) treatment for resistant atopic dermatitis-efficacy and effects on intracellular cytokine levels and CD4 counts. *Acta Derm Venereol* (submitted).

10. Paul C, Lahfa M, Bachelez H, Chevret S, Dubertret L. A randomized controlled evaluator-blinded trial of intravenous immunoglobulin in adults with severe atopic dermatitis. *Br J Dermatol* 2002; **147**: 518–22.

11. Jolles S. A review of high-dose intravenous immunoglobulin (HdIVIg) treatment for atopic dermatitis. *Clin Exp Dermatol* 2002: **27**: 3–7.

12. Grewe M, Bruijnzeel-Koomen C, Schopf E et al. A role for Th1 and Th2 cells in the immunopathogenesis of atopic dermatitis. *Immunol Today* 1998; **19**: 359–61.

13. Bjork L, Andersson U, Chauvet JM, Skansen-Saphir U, Andersson J. Quantification of superantigen induced IFN-γ production by computerized image analysis-inhibition of cytokine production and blast transformation by pooled human IgG. *J Immunol Meth* 1994; **175**: 201–13.

14. Thepen T, Langveld-Wildschut EG, Bihari IC et al. Biphasic response against aeroallergen in atopic dermatitis showing a switch from a

Th2 response to a Th1 response in situ: an immunocytochemical study. *J Allergy Clin Immunol* 1996; **97**: 828–37.

15. Hamid Q, Naseer T, Minshall EM, Song YL, Boguniewicz M, Leung DY. In vivo expression of IL-12 and IL-13 in atopic dermatitis. *J Allergy Clin Immunol* 1996; **98**: 225–31.

16. Trautmann A, Akidis M, Kleeman D et al. T cell-mediated Fas-induced keratinocyte apoptosis plays a key pathogenetic role in eczematous dermatitis. *J Clin Invest* 2000; **106**: 25–35.

17. Haas H, Schlaak M. In vitro synthesis of human IgE is suppressed by human IgG. *J Clin Immunol* 1995; **15**: 172–8.

# Kawasaki disease

**Andrew J Cant and Laura Jones**

**5**

AECA, antiendothelial cell antibodies; ALT, alanine aminotransferase; ANCA, antineutrophil cytosolic antibodies; CRP, C-reactive protein; ESR, erythrocyte sedimentation rate; hdIVIg, high-dose intravenous immunoglobulin; MHC, major histocompatibility complex; PCR, polymerase chain reaction; TGF, transforming growth factor; TNF, tumour necrosis factor; WCC, white cell count.

## Introduction

Kawasaki disease is an acute febrile childhood vasculitic illness that was first described in Japan in the 1960s by Dr Tomasko Kawasaki.[1–3] Since the decline of rheumatoid heart disease, Kawasaki disease is the commonest cause of acquired coronary artery disease in the developed world.

The children described by Kawasaki were mostly less than 5 years of age and had prolonged fever, bilateral non-purulent conjunctivitis, a polymorphus erythematous rash, changes in the oral mucosa, and oedema and redness of the extremities with associated desquamation of the hands and feet. Similar cases were described in the USA in 1971, and it was soon realized that Kawasaki disease occurred worldwide.[4] At the same time it emerged that many patients developed coronary artery abnormalities, detectable on echocardiography. This was associated with a significant mortality rate from acute myocardial infarction. Kawasaki disease has many similarities to the previously recognized condition of infantile periarteritis nodosa, and it is likely that it is not an entirely new entity.

## Epidemiology

Kawasaki disease occurs both in temperate and tropical zones and in urban and rural areas. The highest incidence remains among children of Japanese background. It primarily affects young children, 50% of cases occurring before 2 years of age and 80% by 5 years of age. Recent incidence figures show a rate of 110–150 per 100,000 children aged less than 5 years in Japan, compared to 10 per 100,000 in the USA and 4 per 100,000 in the UK.[5,6] In the USA there is a slightly higher incidence in blacks than in Caucasians.[6] Worldwide there remains a male predominance, and serious complications are also more common in males. Recurrence, defined as a new episode that begins more than 3 months after the platelet count returns to normal, is rare. Recent Japanese studies have reported a recurrence rate of 3%,[7] with a higher recurrence in males and in children who had been less than 2 years of age at the time of their first attack.[8]

## Aetiology

The aetiology of Kawasaki disease has been much debated. The occurrence of clusters of cases has suggested an infective aetiology and many agents have been implicated, including mites, bacteria, spirochaetes, rickettsiae, yersinia, mycoplasma and viruses, including parvovirus, adenovirus, enterovirus, parainfluenza and measles. Recent evidence increasingly suggests that bacterial superantigens provoking a massive inflammatory response cause the typical vasculitic features of Kawasaki disease.[9–11]

## Clinical features

Kawasaki disease is a triphasic illness with acute, subacute and convalescent phases. The acute phase, characterized by fever, conjunctivitis (Fig. 5.1), changes in the oral mucosa and hands and feet, typically lasts 8–15 days without treatment (with a mean of 11 days). In the subacute phase there is desquamation of the palms and soles, arthritis and thrombocytosis which usually lasts until the child is back to normal (approximately 3–4 weeks). It is in the convalescent phase, however, that children are at the greatest risk

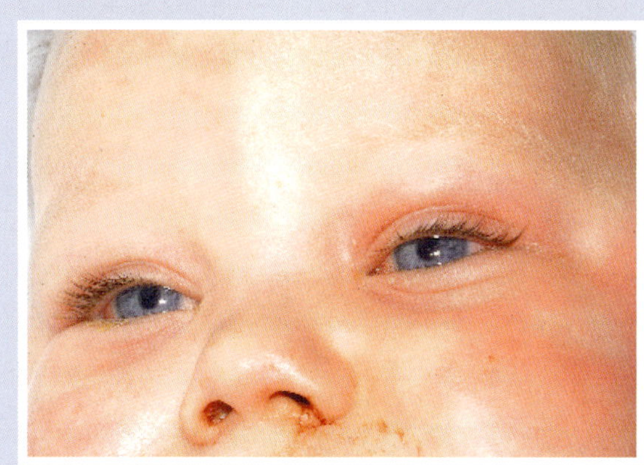



of death from myocardial infarction, following coronary artery occlusion or rupture.

Clinical diagnosis can be difficult, as symptoms may appear sequentially rather than simultaneously, and many features are seen in other conditions. As well as a history of unremitting fever for more than 5 days, changes in the oral mucosa (Fig. 5.2) are the most consistent feature, and are found in 90% of children with Kawasaki disease. Desquamation of the palms and soles is easily recognized but is not a very helpful sign as it occurs relatively late in the illness. The skin rash varies from papular to urticarial and predominantly involves the trunk, but the face and limbs can also be affected and perianal rashes have also been described (Fig. 5.3). Lymphadenopathy is the diagnostic feature reported least often, and is often the sign that is missing in children diagnosed with atypical or incomplete Kawasaki disease. Younger children, especially those below 1 year of age, are more likely to have Kawasaki disease without fulfilling all of the diagnostic criteria. The fever is unresponsive to antipyretics and the child is miserable and inconsolable. The absence of unique clinical features or a single diagnostic test means that diagnosis remains dependent on a high index of suspicion and the use of the diagnostic criteria (Table 5.1). Kawasaki disease is a truly multisystem condition, and less common manifestations are described in Table 5.2. When considering the diagnosis of Kawasaki disease it is important to exclude other illnesses that may present in a similar way (Table 5.3).

An increasing number of infants are being recognized who have atypical or incomplete

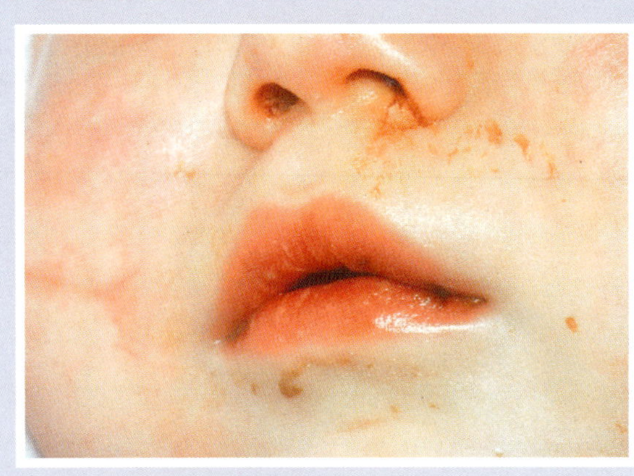

**Fig. 5.2**
*Cracked and fissured lips in patient with Kawasaki disease.*

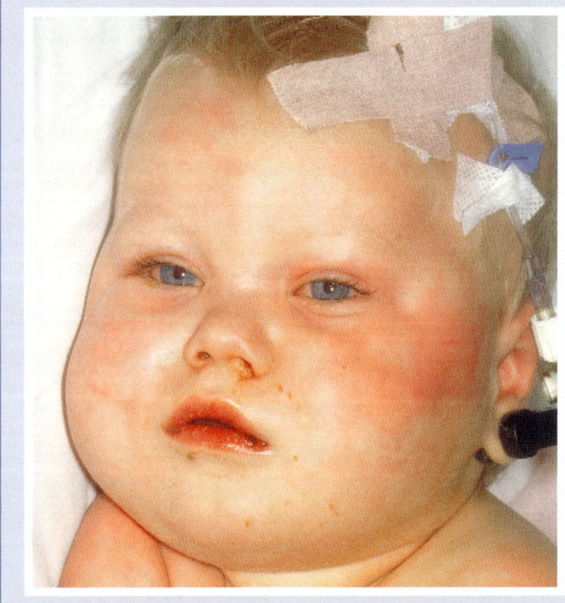

**Fig. 5.3**
*Rash in Kawasaki disease.*

**Table 5.1**
*Diagnostic criteria*

*Presence of at least five of six criteria:*
- *Fever for 5 days or more*
- *Bilateral non-purulent conjunctivitis*
- *Changes in mucous membranes and respiratory tract, e.g. dry reddened cracked lips, strawberry tongue and injected pharynx*
- *Changes in hands and feet – oedema and erythema of palms and soles acutely – desquamation of palms and soles in the convalescent phase*
- *Polymorphus rash*
- *Cervical lymphadenopathy > 1.5 cm in diameter (often unilateral and painful)*

*In the presence of echocardiographically proven coronary arterial aneurysms, the presence of fever and three of the above criteria has been accepted as fulfilling the diagnosis.*

Kawasaki disease but who have gone on to develop coronary artery changes.[12,13]

Cardiological sequelae are the most feared complication of Kawasaki disease, and although early treatment is highly effective in preventing sequelae, they still occur in up to 10% of patients despite treatment. Coronary artery changes may occur within the first 3–14 days of the illness. Pericardial effusions occur in up to 30% of patients in the acute phase and left ventricular dysfunction has been recorded, which has been shown to resolve more quickly in those patients who receive intravenous immunoglobulin.[14] Initially, coronary artery aneurysms develop, but long-term sequelae include arteriosclerosis and coronary artery stenosis, leading to myocardial ischaemia. Myocardial infarction is the principal cause of death.[15–17]

## Laboratory findings

Laboratory investigations can help support a diagnosis of Kawasaki disease but none are diagnostic. Acute-phase proteins (ESR/CRP) are markedly elevated in the acute stages and, if normal, an alternative diagnosis should be considered. $\beta_2$-Microglobulin and $\alpha_1$-antitrypsin are also raised, but will return to normal 8–12 weeks after the onset of the illness. A raised white cell count (granulocytes) is seen in the acute phase, although the well-recognized thrombocytosis is usually not seen until weeks 2 or 3 of the illness. The platelet count rises above 450,000/$\mu$l and can reach 1,000,000/$\mu$l after week 3, and in an uncomplicated course returns to normal 4 weeks after the onset of the disease. Patients may exhibit a normocytic or microcytic anaemia and blood

**Table 5.2**
*Less common features of Kawasaki disease*

- Cough, rhinorrhoea and otitis media
- Abdominal pain, nausea and vomiting
- Obstructive jaundice, splenomegaly and a hydropic gallbladder
- Sterile pyuria and proteinuria
- Lethargy, irritability
- Nerve palsy and aseptic meningitis
- Uveititis
- Swelling and pain of both small and large joints
- Redness and induration at site of previous BCG scar

**Table 5.3**
*Diseases with clinical presentation similar to Kawasaki disease*

- Staphylococcal infection, e.g. scalded skin, toxic shock syndrome
- Streptococcal infection, e.g. scarlet fever
- Viral exanthem, including measles
- Leptospirosis
- Rickettsia infections
- Stevens–Johnson syndrome
- Drug reactions
- Juvenile chronic arthritis

films may demonstrate toxic granulation. Complement component levels, especially C3 and C4, are elevated in the acute phase, as is IgE. Liver enzymes, typically ALT, are often raised and there may also be an elevated bilirubin and reduced serum albumin. A low albumin is a marker of more severe disease.

# Pathology

Although the vasculitis in Kawasaki disease has a predilection for coronary arteries, any vessel in the body can be affected. Aneurysms have been reported in the brachial, renal and iliac vessels, and changes in vessel architecture have been noted in the lung, kidney, pancreas, spleen, gut, mesentery and testes. In the coronary arteries, vasculitis of the microvasculature and major coronary arteries occurs in addition to aneurysm and thrombus formation. Pericarditis, myocarditis, endocarditis and valvulitis can also all occur. Inflammation of the atrioventricular conduction system can lead to arrhythmias (tachycardia and/or bradycardia), which can contribute to intractable cardiac failure.[18,19]

# Bacterial superantigens

Bacterial superantigens, are 20 or 30 kDa proteins with unique immunological properties. Conventional antigens require processing by an antigen-presenting cell such as a macrophage prior to expression in the groove on the inner surface of the MHC class II molecule. T-cell recognition of conventional antigens is highly specific, MHC class II restricted, and typically fewer than 1 in 10,000 T cells will be activated by any particular antigen. Superantigens interact with class II MHC molecules by binding outside the antigen-binding groove to the outer part of the molecule (Fig. 5.4). This abnormal MHC–antigen combination is recognized by the Vβ region on the outer surface of the T-cell receptor. As each T cell belongs to one of only 25 Vβ families, a superantigen can stimulate up to 20% of the T-cell population, depending on the frequency of that specific Vβ population.

Binding to T cells in this way causes proliferation and activation of those cells expressing the specific Vβ regions, with massive release of inflammatory cytokines such as IL-1, IL-2, IFN-γ and TNF-α. Cytokines contribute to the vasculitis and capillary leak, although superantigens themselves may also have a direct toxic effect on the endothelium. Polyclonal B-cell activation leads to antibody production and hypergammaglobulinaemia, autoantibody production (antineutrophil cytosolic antibodies and antiendothelial cell antibodies – ANCA, AECA) and immune complex formation. Recent studies using PCR techniques have reported an increase prevalence of T cells bearing Vβ2 in children with Kawasaki disease, particularly during the second week of illness.[10,11,20]

# Treatment with IVIg

Until the early 1980s aspirin was the initial treatment for Kawasaki disease. This followed trials comparing treatment with aspirin alone against non-steroidal anti-inflammatory agents alone and dipyridamole. The lowest percentage of coronary abnormalities were found in those treated with aspirin alone.[21] However, there are no reported large-scale trials comparing aspirin with placebo.

In the early 1980s IVIg became an established treatment for idiopathic thrombocytopenic purpura (ITP), having been shown to increase significantly the platelet count in cases when there was significant bleeding or a persistently low platelet count. Working on the hypothesis that similar immunological mechanisms were involved in ITP and Kawasaki disease, IVIg was first used in 1982. In 1984 and 1985 Furusho et al.[22] conducted the first randomized trial comparing aspirin treatment alone with aspirin and IVIg. This initial study compared 45 patients treated with aspirin alone against 40 patients treated with aspirin and IVIg; the patients treated with aspirin received 30–50 mg/kg/day while the fever lasted, and then 10–30 g/kg/day. Those treated with IVIg received aspirin at the same dose, plus IVIg at a dose of 0.4 g/kg/day for 5 days.

There was a significant reduction in the frequency of coronary artery dilation and a reduced frequency of persistent dilation in the group treated with IVIg and aspirin, compared to those treated with aspirin alone

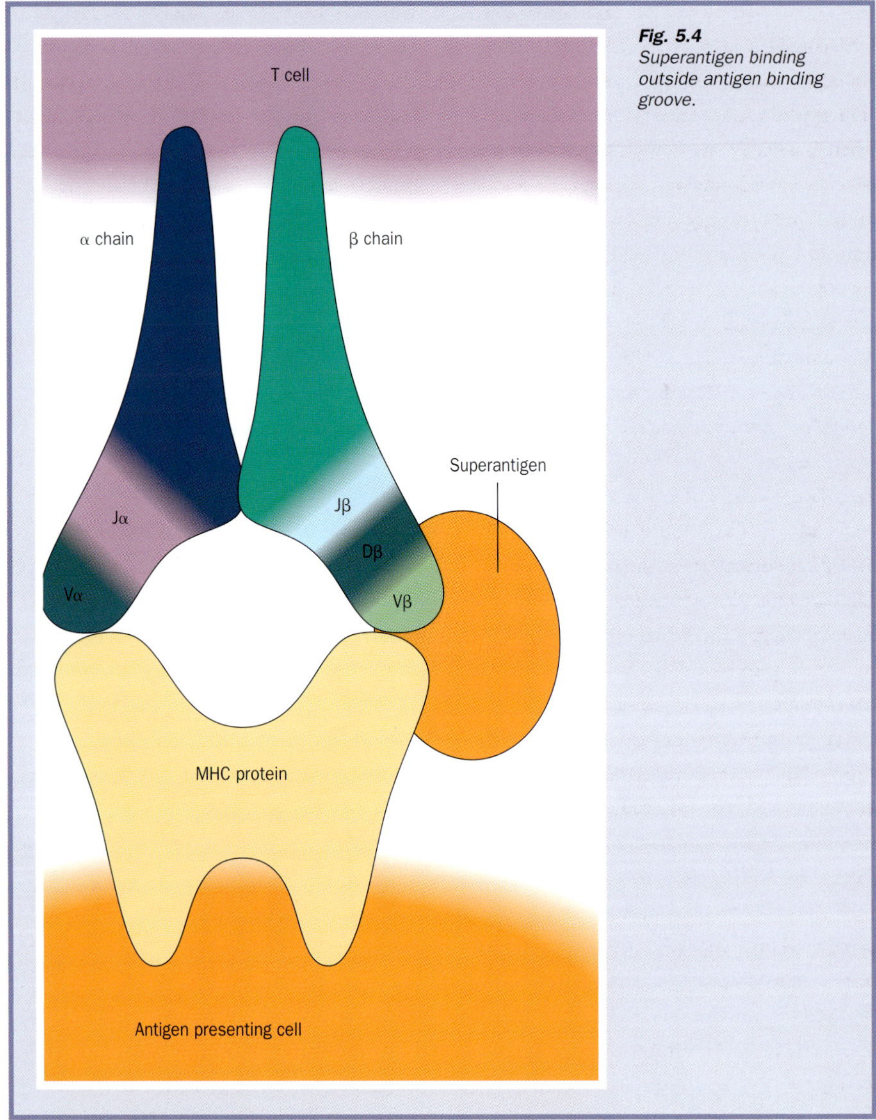


**Fig. 5.4**
*Superantigen binding outside antigen binding groove.*

(15% compared to 42% for the former, and 50% compared to 73% for the latter). There are no studies comparing the effect of IVIg alone with IVIg and aspirin or aspirin alone. There is a widely held belief that aspirin is beneficial as it inhibits platelet aggregation.

In 1986 Newberger et al.[23] published results supporting Furusho's findings. They conducted a multicentre randomized controlled trial looking at 168 children with Kawasaki disease, 84 enrolled into group A (aspirin alone) and 84 into group B (aspirin and IVIg). They achieved 91% follow-up at 2 weeks and 94% follow up at 7 weeks. Excluding the six children who had coronary artery abnormalities at the time of diagnosis, 20% of children treated with aspirin alone, compared to 6.8% of children who also received IVIg, had coronary artery lesions on echocardiography at 2 weeks, and 14.7% and 2.6%, respectively, at 7-week follow-up. The coronary artery abnormalities were most often detected in the left main and left anterior descending arteries and least often in the circumflex artery. Patients also recovered from fever more quickly, temperature falling by 1.3° ($\pm$ 0.16°) between the first and second days of treatment with IVIg and aspirin, compared to 0.42° ($\pm$ 0.11) with aspirin alone. There was also a more rapid decline in WCC and serum $\alpha_1$-antitrypsin in the first 5 days in those treated with IVIg. Platelet counts, however, were similar in both groups.

In 1991 Newberger et al.[24] published data from their 1984–1989 multicentre randomized controlled trial involving 549 children with Kawasaki disease looking at whether single high-dose IVIg (2 g/kg) was as effective as four daily doses of 0.4 g/kg. Children treated with 2 g/kg of IVIg had a shorter duration of fever and a more rapid resolution of inflammatory markers. Of children who received 0.4 g/kg/day of IVIg for 4 days, 29.3% were febrile for at least 3 days after the initial treatment, compared to 19.1% of those treated with 2 g/kg IVIg. At 2 weeks, those treated with single high dose of IVIg had lower CRP and $\alpha_1$-antitrypsin levels and higher serum albumin than those who received the 4-day regimen. In those treated with the 4-day regimen IgG levels on the fourth day of treatment were a strong predictor of outcome, lower levels predicting higher prevalence of coronary artery lesions. In those treated with single-dose HdIVIg there was no correlation.

In 1994, Durongpisitkul et al.[25] published a meta-analysis of 28 studies (24 articles) looking at 4151 patients which supported the view that single high-dose IVIg and aspirin was the most effective way to prevent coronary artery abnormalities. Overall, at 30 days follow-up patients treated with single high-dose IVIg (2 g/kg) had only a 2.3% incidence of coronary artery abnormalities, compared to a 10.3% incidence in those treated with 0.4 g/kg/day of IVIg for 4 days, and 17.3% in those treated with low-dose

IVIg (0.1–0.2 g/kg/day for 5 days). Studies using high and low doses of aspirin were compared in this meta-analysis (> 80 mg/kg/day and < 80 mg/kg/day) but the incidence of coronary artery abnormalities did not appear to be related to aspirin dose.

## Mechanism of action of IVIg

The exact mechanism by which IVIg works in Kawasaki disease remains unclear, but evidence is emerging to support a number of possible actions. In 1981 it was noted that children with ITP treated with IVIg had a marked improvement in their platelet counts. IVIg appeared to block the Fc receptors on phagocytic cells, thereby preventing the removal of 'sensitized' platelets by the liver and spleen. Autoantibody-coated platelets therefore had a prolonged survival.

In addition to Fc receptor blockade, other effects have been demonstrated. Administration of antigen to an animal with an intact immune system will stimulate the production of antibodies; however, if minute amounts of IgG antibodies are administered alongside the antigen no such antibody response occurs.[26] When an antigen binds to a B cell a series of events is initiated, leading to B-cell proliferation and antibody production. When circulating IgG antibodies (e.g. from IVIg) are bound to the antigen, the IgG binds to the Fcγ receptor of the B cell, exerting a negative signal for the B cells, which therefore

do not go on to proliferate and produce antibody. This is the hypothesis behind the reduced levels of platelet antibodies in patients with ITP who have been treated with IVIg. Antibodies also act as antigens (or idiotypes) and promote the production of antibody to antibody or anti-idiotype antibodies. Naturally occurring anti-idiotype antibodies are present in IVIg and some interact with the variable regions of autoantibodies giving IVIg the ability to neutralize autoantibodies, for example anti-factor VIII and ANCA.

Many studies also demonstrate that IVIg can modify cytokine production, increasing production as in the case of TGF-1[27] or decreasing it as in IL-6. Andersson et al.[27] recently suggested that IVIg exerted these changes by affecting antigen-presenting cells and B cells, rather than affecting the T cells directly. In the acute phase of Kawasaki disease TNF-α and IL-6 are both elevated, and Leung et al.[28] have shown that treatment with IVIg reduces levels of both.

IVIg contains high concentrations of specific antibodies which are capable of neutralizing various streptococcal and staphylococcal superantigen toxins. IVIG may limit T-cell proliferation by preventing the binding of these toxins to accompanying cells that would otherwise stimulate T cells. IVIg has also been shown to downregulate complement activation by binding to activated C3b and C4b, thereby preventing their binding to target cells such as the vascular endothelium and so preventing complement-mediated damage. Furthermore, by altering the amount of C3 and C4 in immune complexes, IVIG alters their size and structure and hence their deposition. Both actions may prevent or lessen vasculitis.[29]

## Treatment for unresponsive Kawasaki disease

In 1998 Burns et al.[30] published a retrospective study looking at the outcome for patients who remained febrile and so were retreated with IVIg. In their cohort of 378 patients, 86.81% became and remained afebrile after their first course of treatment with IVIg (2 g/kg). However, 50 children (13.2%) had persistent fever (temperature > 38.3°C throughout IVIg infusion and for 48 hours after its completion) or a recrudescent fever (< 38.3°C for first 48 hours after infusion, but followed by > 38.3°C); 29 (58%) of these patients received further IVIg, in doses of 1 g/kg or 2 g/kg. Patients who had persistent or recrudescent fever had a higher incidence of coronary artery abnormalities. This corroborated their earlier study in 1993.[31]

Despite early treatment with IVIg a minority of patients do not respond.[32,33] Currently there is no consensus on how to treat such patients, but increasingly, further doses of IVIg are being given. Corticosteroids are also being more commonly used in cases of persistent fever, although conclusive data remain scarce, and concern remains about the transient dilatation of coronary arteries during steroid therapy, thereby justifying close echocardiographic monitoring.[34]

There are few data regarding the best treatment for the 3% of patients who relapse, but it appears common practice to treat them with the standard regimens known to be effective in patients who present with the disease for the first time.

Nakamura et al.[35] published data in 1998 looking at cardiac sequelae (coronary aneurysms, coronary artery stenosis, myocardial infarction and valvular lesions) in patients with recurrent disease, and found that they were much more common than in initial presentations. In men, abnormalities occurred in 25.5% of recurrent cases compared to 14.9% of initial cases; and in women, in 16.1% of recurrent cases compared to 9.8% initial cases.

## Side-effects of IVIg

Although IVIg is now widely used, occasional side-effects do occur and should not be forgotten. Common but minor side-effects include a rash (often macular and polymorphous), fever and headache, the latter occurring in 1–15% of patients. Rarer side effects include aseptic meningitis. Transmission of bloodborne pathogens is limited by checks on plasma donors and the strict sterilization procedures and the viral inactivation that IVIg is subjected to, which reduces the risk of viral transmission to a very low level. Nevertheless, a very small risk of infection with agents such as hepatitis C cannot be entirely eliminated.

## Patients who do not fulfil diagnostic criteria

The clinical criteria required for a diagnosis of Kawasaki disease were summarized by the American Heart Association in 1993 and are listed in Table 5.1. Increasingly since then, Kawasaki disease has been both diagnosed and treated in a large number of children who do not strictly fulfil the AHA criteria. Witt et al.[12] in a retrospective study covering the years 1991–1997, found that it was children under 1 year old who were most likely to be diagnosed and treated without fulfilling all of the criteria. However, it was also these children who were most at risk of developing coronary artery abnormalities. Interestingly, these patients also had higher platelet counts and lower haematocrit levels than controls. Over a 7-year period 127 patients were reviewed, all of whom received treatment with IVIG: 81 (64%) met the criteria and 46 (36%) did not. However, of those who went on to develop coronary artery aneurysms, 60% had not fulfilled the AHA criteria. Stockhein et al.[36] also highlighted the

difficulty of diagnosing Kawasaki disease in older children, especially those over the age of 8. Older children appear to be diagnosed later, and the authors surmised that this is possibly because less typical signs of Kawasaki disease, such as abdominal pain and arthritis, were more common.

Much debate remains about IVIg treatment for children who do not strictly fulfil the criteria. At present the balance of opinion contends that treatment is relatively safe and effective, although expensive, and although some children who do not have Kawasaki disease may be treated unnecessarily, others with Kawasaki disease will be treated when otherwise they would not have been. If this prevents a significant amount of coronary artery disease, then this strategy is probably worthwhile.

## Long-term sequelae

Most children with Kawasaki disease make a full recovery from the acute illness. Untreated, up to 20% of patients develop coronary artery abnormalities; if early IVIg treatment is given coronary artery abnormalities occur in between 4 and 8% of children.[37–39] Echocardiography is a sensitive and practical method of detecting such abnormalities. Follow-up studies have shown that patients with normal or only minimal coronary artery changes at the time of the acute illness, and normal echocardiographs at 6-month follow-up, require no further intervention or follow-up. Small and medium-sized arterial aneurysms diagnosed at the time of illness may regress spontaneously, but any aneurysm remaining visible on echocardiography at 6 months' follow-up warrants further investigation with imaging such as angiography. Patients with giant arterial aneurysms are at significant risk of developing coronary artery stenosis and consequent myocardial ischaemia.[16,39] More recent data have highlighted a concern that even in patients in whom the coronary artery abnormalities regress, the arteries may remain abnormal – thickened and poorly contractile – thereby increasing the risk of atherosclerotic disease at an early age.

In older children, non-invasive tests such as dobutamine stress echocardiography and exercise tests may help in assessing the risks of impending ischaemic damage. For patients with persistent coronary artery abnormalities, anticoagulation and antiplatelet treatments are advocated, and active measures to reduce other risk factors such as hyperlipidaemia and smoking are also encouraged.

Long-term dermatological sequelae may occur. Eberhard et al.[40] described 10 patients developing psoriatic skin eruptions during the acute and convalescent phases of Kawasaki disease, and 11% of another series of patients developed re-peeling of the skin, some for several years after their episode of Kawasaki disease. There were no long-term sequelae following re-peeling, and the mechanism for the re-peeling was unclear.[41]

Kawasaki disease remains a clinically significant and intriguing childhood illness: diagnosis still relies on clinical acumen and the use of diagnostic criteria. The current recommendations for treatment of Kawasaki disease are shown in Table 5.4. A series of well

**Table 5.4**
*Current recommendations*

- *hdIVIg 2 g/kg over 12 hours, within the first 10 days of illness*
- *Aspirin 80–100 mg/kg/day in four divided doses in acute phase*
- *Monitor salicylate levels*
- *Aspirin 3–5 mg/kg/day in a single dose in convalescent phase. Continue for 6–12 weeks if no coronary abnormality, longer term if coronary abnormalities have occurred*
- *Other agents:*
  - *Dipyridamole (3–4 mg/kg/day in three doses)*
  - *Corticosteroids*
  - *Repeat doses of IVIg*
  - *Anticoagulation*
- *Recommended imaging: ECG and echocardiogram at diagnosis, at 3–6 weeks and at 3–6 months*

conducted, large randomized controlled trials has shown high-dose IVIg to be of dramatic proven benefit. This remains the mainstay of treatment, along with aspirin. However, it should be remembered that despite treatment cardiological sequelae can occur.

## References


1. Kawasaki T. Acute febrile mucocutaneous syndrome with lymphoid involvement with specific desquamation of fingers and toes in children. [Japanese] *Jpn J Allergy* 1967; **116:** 178–222.

2. Kawasaki T, Koraski F, Ohawa S, Shigematsu I, Yangara H. A new infantile acute febrile mucocutaneous lymph node syndrome (MLNS) prevailing in Japan. *Pediatrics* 1974; **54:** 271–6.

3. Kawasaki T. Mucocutaneous lymph node syndrome. *Acta Pathol Japon* 1982; **32:** 63–72.

4. Morens DM, Melish ME. Kawasaki disease. In: Feigin RD, Cherry JC, eds. *Textbook of Pediatric Infectious Diseases.* Philadelphia: WB Saunders, 1998.

5. Yanagawa H, Nakamura Y, Yashiro M et al. Incidence survey of Kawasaki disease in 1997 and 1998 in Japan. *Pediatrics* 2001; **107:** E33.

6. Karyl S, Barron S, Stanford T et al. Report of the National Institutes of Health Workshop on Kawasaki disease. *J Rheumatol* 1999; **26:** 170–90.

7. Yanagawa H, Nakamura Y, Yashiro M et al. Update of the epidemiology of Kawasaki disease from results of 1993–94 nationwide survey. *J Epidemiol* 1996; **6:** 148–57.

8. Nakamura Y, Hirose K, Yanagawa H, Kato H, Kawasaki T. Incidence rate of recurrent Kawasaki disease in Japan. *Acta Pediatr* 1994; **83:** 1061–4.

9. Johnson HM, Russell JK, Pontzer CH. Superantigens in human disease. *Sci Am* 1992; April: 40–73.

10. Curtis N, Zherg R, Lamb JR, Levin M. Evidence for a superantigenic mediated process in Kawasaki disease. *Arch Dis Child* 1995; **72;** 308–11.

11. Curtis N, Levin M. Superantigen diseases. *Rec Adv Pediatr* 1986; **15:** 31–51.

12. Witt MT, Minich LL, Bohnsack JF, Young PC. Kawasaki disease; more patients are being diagnosed who do not meet American Heart Association criteria. *Pediatrics* 1999; **104:** E10.

13. Fukushige J, Takahashi N, Ueda Y, Ueda K. Incidence and clinical features of incomplete Kawasaki disease. *Acta Pediatr* 1994; **83:** 1057–60.

14. Moran AM, Newberger JW, Sanders SP et al. Abnormal myocardial mechanics in Kawasaki disease: rapid response to gammaglobulin. *Am Heart J* 2000; **139:** 217–23.

15. Sasaguri Y, Kato H. Regression of aneurysms in Kawasaki disease: a pathological study. *J Pediatr* 1982; **100:** 225–31.

16. Kato H, Ichinose E, Kawasaki T. Myocardial infarction in Kawasaki disease: clinical analyses in 195 cases. *J Paediatr* 1986; **108:** 923–7.

17. Dajani AS, Tabert KA, Gerber MA et al. Special report: Diagnosis and therapy of Kawasaki disease in children. *Circulation* 1993; **87:** 1176–80.

18. Fujiwara H, Hamashima Y. Pathology of the heart in Kawasaki disease. *Pediatrics* 1978; **61:** 100–7.

19. Gidding SS, Shulman ST, Ilbawi M, Crussi F, Duffy CE. Mucocutaneous lymph node syndrome (Kawasaki disease): delayed aortic and mitral insufficiency secondary to active valvulitis. *J Am Coll Cardiol* 1987; **7**: 894–7.

20. Curtis N, Levin M. Kawasaki disease thirty years on. *Curr Opin Paediatr* 1998; **10**: 24–33.

21. Kato H, Kaike S, Tokayam T. Kawasaki disease: effect of treatment on coronary artery involvement. *Pediatrics* 1979, **63**: 175–9.

22. Furusho K, Nakano H, Sinomiya K et al. High dose intravenous immunoglobulin for Kawasaki disease. *Lancet* 1984; **ii**: 1055–8.

23. Newberger J, Takahashi M, Burns JC et al. The treatment of Kawasaki syndrome with intravenous gamma globulin. *N Engl J Med* 1986; **315**: 341–7.

24. Newberger JW, Takahashi M, Beiser AS et al. A single intravenous infusion of gamma globulin as compared with four infusions in the treatment of acute Kawasaki syndrome. *N Engl J Med* 1991; **324**: 633–9.

25. Durongpistkul K, Guraraj V, Park JM, Martin CF. The prevention of coronary artery aneurysm in Kawasaki disease: a meta-analysis on the efficacy of aspirin and immunoglobulin treatment. *Paediatrics* 1995; **95**: 1057–61.

26. Fridman WH, Teillaird JH, Sautes C. Role of Fc receptors in immunomodulation by intravenous therapy. In: Kazatchine MD, Morell A, eds. *Intravenous Immunoglobulin: Research and Therapy*. New York: Parthenon, 1996.

27. Andersson J, Norrby-Teglund A, Kotb M et al. Modulation of the cytokine network by intravenous immunoglobulin. In: Kazatchine MD, Morell A, eds. *Intravenous Immunoglobulin: Research and Therapy*. New York: Parthenon, 1996.

28. Leung DYM. Clinical relevance of superantigens and their in viro response to intravenous immunoglobulin therapy. In: Kazatchine MD, Morell A, eds. *Intravenous Immunoglobulin: Research and Therapy*. New York: Parthenon, 1996.

29. Kazatchine MD. Mechanisms of action of intravenous immunoglobulin in immune-mediated diseases. In: Kazatchine MD, Morell A eds. *Intravenous Immunoglobulin Research and Therapy*. New York: Parthenon, 1996.

30. Burns JC, Capparelli EV, Brown JA, Newberger JW. Intravenous gammaglobulin treatment and re-treatment in Kawasaki disease. *Pediatr Infect Dis J* 1998; **17**: 1144–8.

31. Sundel RP, Burns JC, Baker A et al. Gammaglobulin re-treatment in Kawasaki disease. *J Pediatr* 1993; **123**: 657–9.

32. Han, RK, Silverman ED, Newman A, McCrindle BW. Management and outcome of persistent or recurrent fever after initial intravenous gamma globulin therapy in acute Kawasaki disease. *Arch Pediatr Adolesc Med* 2000; **154**: 694–9.

33. Fukunishi M, Kikkawa M, Hamaia K et al. Prediction of non responsiveness to intravenous high dose gammaglobulin therapy in patients with Kawasaki disease at onset. *J Pediatr* 2000; **137**: 172–6.

34. Hashino K, Ishii M, Iemura M, Akagi T, Kato H. Re-treatment for immune globulin-resistant Kawasaki disease: a comparative study of additional immune globulin and steroid pulse therapy. *Paediatr Int* 2001; **43**: 211–17.

35. Nakamura Y, Yanagawa H, Ojima T, Kawasaki T, Kato H. Cardiac sequelae of Kawasaki disease among recurrent cases. *Arch Dis Child* 1998; **78**: 163–5.

36. Stockhein JA, Innocentini N, Shulman ST.

Kawasaki disease in elder children and adolescents. *J Pediatr* 2000; **137**: 250–2.

37. Melish ME, Hicks RV. Kawasaki syndrome: clinical features, pathophysiology, etiology and therapy. *J Rheumatol* 1990; **17** (Suppl 24): 2–9.

38. Nakamura Y, Fujita Y, Nagai M et al. Cardiac sequelae of Kawasaki disease in Japan: statistical analysis. *Paediatrics* 1991; **88**: 1144–7.

39. Yanagawa H, Nakamura Y, Sakata K, Yashiro M. Use of intravenous globulin for Kawasaki disease: effects on cardiac sequelae. Paediatr Cardiol 1997; **18**: 19–23.

40. Eberhard BA, Sundes RP, Newberger JW et al. Psoriatic eruption in Kawasaki disease. *J Pediatr* 2000; **137**: 578–80.

41. Michie C, Kinsler V, Tulloh R, Davidson S. Recurrent skin peeling following Kawasaki disease. *Arch Dis Child* 2000; **83**: 353–5.

# Toxic epidermal necrolysis

## Nicholas M Craven

EM, erythema multiforme; MHC, major histocompatibility syndrome; TNF, tumour necrosis factor

## Introduction

Toxic epidermal necrolysis (TEN) and Stevens–Johnson syndrome (SJS) are rare, rapidly evolving and potentially life-threatening skin reactions, usually resulting from an adverse drug reaction. The term 'toxic epidermal necrolysis' was first coined by Lyell in 1956.[1] The original paper described four patients who developed skin loss with the appearance of scalding. It subsequently became clear that these initial cases represented two different conditions, 'true' TEN and staphylococcal scalded skin syndrome. In 1922 Stevens and Johnson had described two children with conjunctivitis, stomatitis and a cutaneous eruption.[2] As further cases emerged, it became apparent that SJS could progress to a stage indistinguishable from TEN, and most authors now consider these conditions to be different points on the same spectrum of this cutaneous reaction pattern.

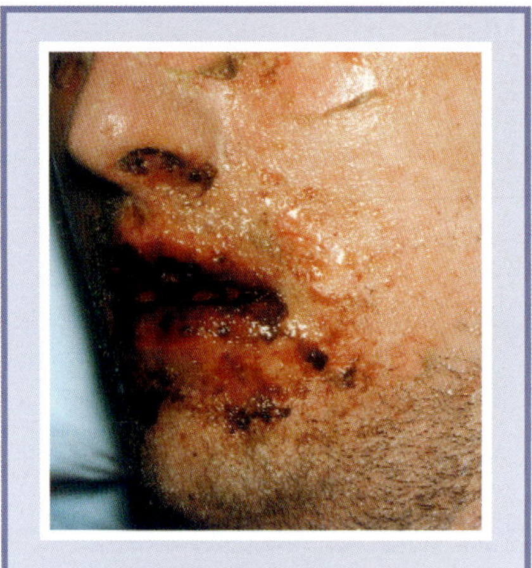

**Fig. 6.1**
*Haemorrhagic crusting of the lips in a patient with toxic epidermal necrolysis.*

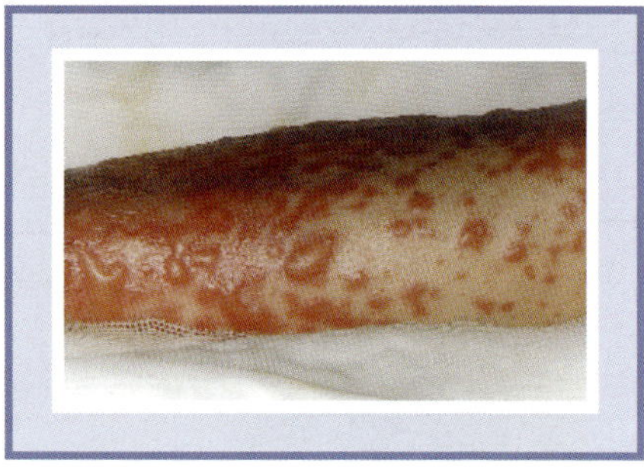

**Fig. 6.2**
*Haemorrhagic blistering macules on the limb of a patient with toxic epidermal necrolysis.*

TEN and SJS are characterized by the development of full-thickness epidermal necrosis with involvement of mucosal surfaces (Fig. 6.1), and are distinguished arbitrarily on the basis of extent of cutaneous involvement. The primary cutaneous lesions of TEN and SJS are usually irregular, atypical 'two-zone' flat target lesions, in contrast to the typical three-zone target lesions of erythema multiforme (EM), or flat purpuric macules, either of which can develop central blistering as the necrotic epidermis separates from the underlying dermis (Fig. 6.2). These lesions preferentially involve the trunk, face, flexures and proximal limbs. Confluence of primary lesions produces areas of widespread epidermal detachment with a positive Nikolsky sign, the development of flaccid blisters or frank epidermal loss (Fig. 6.3). In TEN there is epidermal loss of 30% or more of body surface area; in SJS 10% or less, with cases of 10–30% epidermal loss being classified as TEN–SJS overlap. Rarely, TEN develops as confluent areas of erythema without discrete targets or macules (TEN 'without spots').[3] EM major (EM with mucosal involvement) should be distinguished from SJS/TEN in view of its different aetiologies and prognosis[4] (Table 6.1).

Both conditions are rare. The incidence of TEN is approximately 0.4–1.2 cases per $10^6$ population per annum, and that of SJS 1–6 cases per $10^6$ population per annum.[5] The great majority of cases of TEN/SJS can be attributed to drugs. Although all ages are affected, the condition becomes more common with increasing age (probably

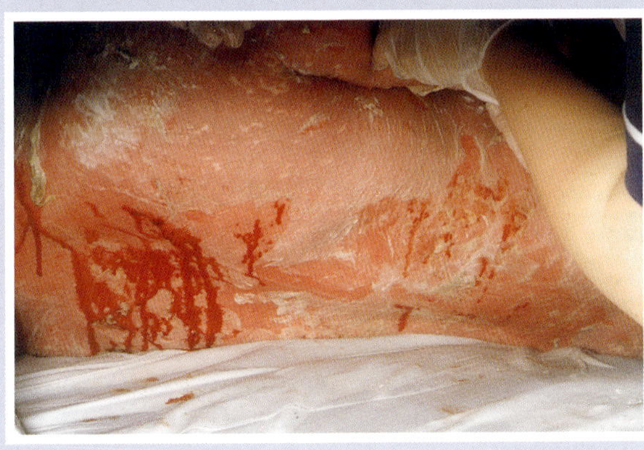

**Fig. 6.3**
Toxic epidermal necrolysis with extensive loss of epidermis from the back.

**Table 6.1**
Classification of EM, SJS and TEN*

| Category | Skin lesions | Mucosal lesions | Extent of epidermal detachment |
|---|---|---|---|
| **EM minor** | Typical targets or raised atypical targets in predominantly acral distribution | No | Virtually none |
| **EM major** | Typical targets or raised atypical targets in predominantly acral distribution | Yes | Usually <10% |
| **SJS** | Macules or flat atypical targets, blisters, predominantly central and flexural distribution | Yes | <10% |
| **SJS–TEN overlap** | Macules or flat atypical targets, confluent erythema, blisters, Nikolsky +ve, widespread distribution | Yes | 10–30% |
| **TEN** | Macules or flat atypical targets, confluent erythema, blisters, Nikolsky +ve, widespread distribution | Yes | >30% |
| **TEN 'without spots'** | Confluent erythema, blisters, Nikolsky +ve, widespread distribution | Yes | >10% |

EM, erythema multiforme; SJS, Stevens–Johnson syndrome; TEN, toxic epidermal necrolysis.
*Adapted from Bastuji-Garin S, Rzany B, Stern RS et al. Arch Dermatol 1993; **129:** 92–6.[3]

reflecting greater use of medications). In a recent large study, the commonest culprit drugs were sulphonamides, with rates of up to 4.5 cases per million users per week. Other frequently implicated drugs included anticonvulsant agents, non-steroidal anti-inflammatories (particularly oxicams), allopurinol, chlormezanone and corticosteroids.[5] The incidence of TEN in HIV-positive patients is about one case per $10^3$ population per annum, possibly reflecting the associated immunological dysfunction[6] in addition to the higher prevalence of medication use in this group. A higher than expected incidence of TEN is seen in systemic lupus erythematosus, graft versus host disease,[7] and in patients treated for brain tumours or head injury. Exceptionally TEN has been attributed to infections such as *Mycoplasma pneumoniae* and herpes simplex virus. In rare cases no cause can be found.[8]

The mortality of TEN is approximately 30% and that of SJS is below 5%.[9] Survivors are at risk of scarring from mucosal involvement: 40–50% develop ocular complications, including keratoconjunctivitis sicca, conjunctival squamous metaplasia, corneal pannus and blindness. Involvement of the tracheal, oesophageal, anal and genital mucosae can lead to the development of strictures.[10]

# Pathogenesis

Although the pathogenesis of TEN remains uncertain, accumulating evidence suggests that drugs or drug metabolites act as haptens bound to epidermal proteins[11] and stimulate a cell-mediated immune response in patients with a particular genetic predisposition. A significant association of TEN with HLA B12 has been demonstrated, with other HLA phenotypes linked to particular culprit drugs.[12] Most patients with sulphonamide-induced TEN are slow acetylators;[13] defects in the detoxification of culprit drug metabolites have been found in patients with sulphonamide- or anticonvulsant-induced TEN, and in their first-degree relatives.[14,15] The evidence suggesting a cell-mediated response includes a report of positive patch and intradermal tests to culprit drugs,[16] and the nature of the inflammatory infiltrate within lesional skin. CD4$^+$ lymphocytes predominate in lesional dermis,[14,17] whereas CD8$^+$ cells predominate in lesional epidermis[14,18,19] and are also found in blister fluid.[20] Cells of the monocyte–macrophage lineage are found within both dermis and epidermis.[14,21] TNF-α is present in lesional epidermis[21] and within blister fluid. Keratinocytes express HLA-DR[17] and ICAM-1,[22] indicating interaction with activated T cells.[23]

Keratinocytes in lesional skin undergo apoptosis.[24] This complex process of programmed cell death has several recognized triggers: TNF and cytotoxic T lymphocytes are both triggers of apoptosis in target cells. One of the best-studied of the apoptosis signalling pathways is the interaction between Fas (CD95) and its ligand (FasL).[25] Fas is a member of the TNF receptor gene superfamily and is normally expressed on the surface of keratinocytes. In patients with TEN, keratinocytes also express lytically active FasL, which plays a major role in the induction of apoptosis in the target keratinocytes.[26] There is some evidence suggesting involvement of the perforin–granzyme apoptosis pathway in the pathogenesis of SJS.[27,28] The extent of the role played by this and other pathways of apoptosis in the spectrum of TEN and SJS is not yet clear.

## Management of TEN and SJS

In patients presenting with a typical picture of TEN or SJS a confident clinical diagnosis can usually be made. Nevertheless, a biopsy should be taken of an affected area of skin to exclude conditions that can be confused with TEN/SJS, such as staphylococcal scalded skin syndrome or paraneoplastic pemphigus. Prompt discontinuation of causative drugs has been shown to improve the prognosis.[29] However, identification of the causative drug can be difficult, and as yet no completely reliable tests are available that will identify the culprit from a list of possible candidates. As a general rule, drugs that have been commenced in the 4 weeks before the onset of symptoms are usually responsible.[5] In practice, if any doubt persists, all drugs should be stopped if possible.

## Supportive treatment

The main cause of death from TEN and SJS is infection; less common causes include gastrointestinal haemorrhage, pulmonary embolism, respiratory failure and renal failure.[10] The mainstay of treatment at the present time remains supportive therapy aimed at reducing the risk of these complications by replacement of lost fluids, maintaining a warm environment to reduce heat loss, the use of topical antiseptic preparations to reduce colonization of the skin with potentially pathogenic organisms, and regular monitoring for sepsis.[30] It is generally recommended, therefore, that such patients should be treated in a unit familiar with managing widespread skin loss and the associated medical complications, such as a burns unit or appropriate high-dependency unit.

## Prevention of disease progression

A number of different treatments have been

tried in an attempt to arrest the progression of the epidermal loss that characterizes these conditions.[31] The use of systemic steroids in TEN and SJS is widespread but remains controversial. Several reports suggest that steroids increase morbidity and mortality, usually by increasing the risk of sepsis.[32,33] Guibal et al.[34] reported a number of cases of TEN occurring in patients already taking high-dose steroids. In these patients the onset of TEN appeared to be delayed following exposure to the culprit drug, but the progression of disease was not halted.[34] In contrast, there are a number of case reports and short studies advocating the use of high-dose steroids early in the evolution of these conditions.[35–37] It is possible, therefore, that the early use of high-dose steroids may prove beneficial in aborting further epithelial loss in patients with evolving TEN or SJS; this needs to be tested in a randomized controlled trial. It is, however, generally accepted that continued administration of steroids is counterproductive once extensive skin loss has occurred.

There are several reports of small numbers of patients with TEN treated with other potential disease-modifying treatments. Heng and Allen[19] reported five patients with TEN: four survived following treatment with cyclophosphamide 100–300 mg daily, and steroids (prednisolone 60–120 mg or methylprednisolone 1 g daily). The fifth died, having had supportive treatment only.[19]

Arévalo et al.[38] reported an improved outcome in 11 consecutive patients with TEN treated with cyclosporin 3 mg/kg/day compared to six historical controls treated with cyclophosphamide and steroids. Egan et al.[39] report a beneficial response to plasmapheresis in a retrospective study of 16 patients. *N*-acetylcysteine and pentoxifylline have both been used with apparent success in small numbers of patients.[40,41] The only controlled trial undertaken so far is of thalidomide, selected as a potent inhibitor of tumour necrosis factor-$\alpha$ (a cytokine implicated in the pathogenesis of TEN). The trial was stopped early, with mortality in the treatment arm being significantly higher than that in the placebo arm.[42]

## Intravenous immunoglobulins

Intravenous immunoglobulin (IVIg) is a heterogeneous product derived from pooled human plasma, and has demonstrated therapeutic benefit in a wide variety of conditions.[43] Among the many biological effects attributed to IVIg several could theoretically be beneficial in patients with TEN/SJS: modulation of immune activity of both CD4$^+$ and CD8$^+$ cells owing to the presence of antibodies directed against T-cell surface molecules, such as the T-cell receptor, CD4 and MHC; inhibition of phagocytosis by competing for Fc receptor binding on phagocytic cells; alteration of cytokine profiles attributed to the presence of antibodies directed against IL-1, TNF, IL-6 and members of the interferon family;[43] and prevention of interaction between Fas and FasL owing to the presence of naturally occurring Fas-blocking antibodies.[26] The anti-infective properties of immunoglobulins may help to reduce colonization and the risk of secondary infection (without promoting resistance, which occurs with the prophylactic use of antibiotics). In addition, replacement of intravascular fluid and protein, with its associated oncotic effect, may be an important non-specific role of IVIg in these patients, who become severely hypovolaemic and hypoalbuminaemic through greatly increased loss of fluid and protein via the exposed dermis, and reduced albumin production.

IVIG is not without potential risks. A review of 480 infusions of high-dose IVIg in 83 patients with idiopathic thrombocytopenic purpura (ITP) reported side-effects occurring in 4% of cases. Headache was the most commonly reported problem; more severe adverse reactions included aseptic meningitis (14 cases), renal dysfunction (12 cases, with one case of acute renal failure), haemolytic anaemia (eight cases), anaphylactic/oid reaction caused by too rapid an infusion rate (three cases), and severe skin reactions (one severe case, described as EM, with 80% body surface involvement of iris lesions, vesicles, bullae and epidermal necrosis; and one case of purpuric erythema).[44,45] As the product is

pooled from multiple donors there is a risk of transmission of infection, although this is minimized by careful selection of donors, screening of plasma for known infection, and removal/inactivation procedures during the production process.

Amato et al.[46] first reported the use of high-dose IVIg in the treatment of a 22–month-old girl who had developed SJS following phenobarbitol. However, high-dose systemic steroids were given concurrently, making it difficult to attribute the patient's recovery specifically to the use of IVIG. A number of subsequent case reports detailing patients with SJS or TEN responding to various IVIg regimens are summarized in Table 6.2.

The observation that Fas–Fas-ligand interaction is a major trigger for keratinocyte apoptosis in TEN[26] has prompted further recent interest in the use of high-dose IVIg. A series of elegant *in vitro* studies demonstrated a protective effect of IVIg against Fas-mediated apoptosis, owing to the presence of naturally occurring anti-Fas immunoglobulin, which acts to inhibit binding of Fas with its ligand.[26] This was followed by an open, non-controlled study of the use of IVIg *in vivo*. Ten patients (six male, four female; mean age 39.4 years, range 11–88) with a diagnosis of TEN (mean area of epidermal loss 28.5%; range 5–60%) were recruited across three centres and were treated with IVIg at doses ranging from 0.2 to 0.75 g/kg/day for 4

**Table 6.2**
IVIg in SJS and TEN

| Author (ref) | Number of patients | Diagnosis (no. of pts) | IVIg dose | Other systemic treatment | Outcome | Comments |
|---|---|---|---|---|---|---|
| Amato et al.[46] | 1 | SJS | 5 g/day × 9 doses | Steroids† | Survived | |
| Moudgil et al.[52] | 2 | SJS | 0.4 g/kg/day × 4 days (1 pt); 2 g/kg × 1 dose (1 pt) | | Survived | |
| Sanwo et al.[53] | 2 | SJS (1) ED (1) | 0.4 g/kg/day × 5 days | | Survived | Both patients had AIDS |
| Viard et al.[26] | 10 | TEN | 0.2 – 0.75 g/kg/day × 4 days | | All survived | |
| Phan et al.[54] | 1 | TEN | 0.4 g/kg × 2 doses | | | Patient had AIDS |
| Straussberg et al.[55] | 1 | SJS / AHS | 0.5 g/kg × 4 days | Steroids† | Survived | |
| Magina et al.[56] | 1 | TEN | 0.4 g/kg/day × 5 days | | Survived | |
| Eisen et al.[57] | 1 | TEN | 0.75 g/kg/day × 4 days | | Survived | |
| Morici et al.[47] | 12 (7 treated with IVIg) | SJS | 1.5–2 g/kg (single infusion) | | All survived | 2/12 treated with steroids; 3/12 supportive measures only |
| Paquet et al.[58] | 1 | TEN | 0.75 g/kg/day × 5 days | Steroids§ | Survived | |
| Brett et al.[59] | 1 | SJS | 1 g/kg/day (2 doses) | Steroids§ | Survived | |
| Corne et al.[60] | 1 | TEN | 0.4 g/kg/day × 5 days | N-acetyl cysteine† | Survived | |
| Stella et al.[48] | 9 | SJS (1) TEN (8) | 0.6–0.7 g/kg/day × 4 days | Steroids† | 8/9 survived | 3 cases of respiratory failure and 1 renal failure among survivors. High incidence of malignancy. |
| Prins et al.[49] | 48 | SJS/TEN overlap (10) TEN (38) | 0.2–2.9 g/kg/day × 1–5 days | Steroids§ (25% of cases) | 42/48 survived | Multicentre study |
| Bachot et al.[50] | 34 | SJS (9) SJS/TEN overlap (5) TEN (20) | 2 g/kg total dose over 2 to 5 days | | 23/34 survived | Single centre. Nephrotoxic effect of IVIg noted. No difference in mortality from that predicted by disease severity score |

SJS, Steven–Johnson syndrome; TEN, toxic epidermal necrolysis; ED, erythroderma; AHS, anticonvulsant hypersensitivity syndrome.
†used concurrently with IVIg;  § used prior to IVIg.

consecutive days. Mean delay between onset of TEN and treatment with IVIg was 3.6 days (range 2–5). The progression of skin disease halted within 24–48 hours after IVIg infusion. This was followed by rapid healing of the skin (mean 6.9 days; range 4–12) and the survival of all 10 patients.[26]

Morici et al.[47] reviewed their use of IVIg in the treatment of children with SJS. Seven of 12 children (mean age 7.5 years; range 4–13) with SJS were treated with IVIg at a dose of 1.5–2 g/kg as a single infusion. Mean delay between admission and IVIg treatment was 3 days (range 1–8). One of these children was excluded from further study because of underlying lung disease. The other children (means age 6.4 years; range 0.8–17) were treated with corticosteroids (2) or supportive care only (3). Treatments were not randomized, and the reasons for choosing treatment regimens are not stated. The duration of fever and hospitalization was reduced in the IVIg-treated group, but statistical significance was marginal. All the patients survived. It is possible that several of the children reported here could be classified as having erythema multiforme major rather than SJS.

Stella et al.[48] reported their experience with IVIg in the management of nine patients with TEN and SJS (mean age 54 years, range 27–68; mean area of epidermal detachment 16%, range 4–37%). IVIg was administered at a dose of 0.6–0.7 g/kg/day for four successive days. In addition, patients were treated with intravenous methylprednisolone 250 mg 6–hourly for 48 hours. Of the nine treated patients, eight survived. Epidermal loss continued for an average of 4.8 days from the onset of IVIG therapy (range 3–10 days). Complete healing took an average of 12 days (range 7–17). Three of the survivors suffered respiratory failure during the course of their disease, requiring ventilation, and one developed renal failure requiring dialysis. A surprisingly high number of these patients had preceding malignancy (78%), usually associated with a higher risk of mortality with TEN.

The largest relevant trial to date is an open study of the outcome from TEN and SJS/TEN overlap in 48 consecutive patients treated with IVIg at 14 centres.[49] IVIG was administered at a dose of 0.2–2.9 (mean 0.7) g/kg/day for 1–5 (mean 4) consecutive days, in addition to standard supportive therapy; 25% of patients had received oral or intravenous steroids prior to the initiation of IVIg infusion. Overall survival at 45 days was 87.5% (42/48). Factors associated with a better prognosis include younger age (mean age of survivors 39.6 years vs 66.2 years for patients who died), lower extent of skin loss (mean area of epidermal loss in survivors 42% vs 65%), and a lower incidence of underlying disease (renal and cardiovascular insufficiency, hypertension, infectious disease and cancer all more frequent in those who died). Non-significant trends were seen with regard to benefit from the earlier administration of IVIg (mean delay to IVIg in survivors 6.8 days vs 10.2 days) and total dose of IVIg given (mean dose of IVIg in survivors 2.8 g/kg vs 2 g/kg). No severe side effects were reported with IVIg infusion. The study also reported variability in the Fas-blocking effect in different batches of commercially available preparations of IVIg, although this did not correlate with response to treatment in the few patients whose IVIg was assessed in this manner.

Bachot et al.[50] report an open study of the outcome of 34 patients treated with IVIg. Based at a single centre, the patients (20 with TEN, 9 with SJS and 5 with SJS–TEN overlap) were treated with IVIg at a dose of 2 g/kg over 2–5 days. Using a validated score of disease severity (SCORTEN)[51] they predicted a mortality of 24% (8.2 deaths) in this cohort of patients. The actual mortality was 32% (11 deaths). Increased mortality was observed mainly in those over 70 years of age (seven deaths vs three predicted). Importantly, they did not observe any slowing of the progression of epidermal loss. Indeed, in patients treated earlier in the course of their disease, epidermal loss progressed more than in those treated later. A decrease in renal function was noted suggesting a nephrotoxic effect of high-dose IVIg. Although commenting that their results do not exclude a weak benefit on mortality, they concluded

that IVIG cannot be considered the standard therapy for TEN, and should be discouraged in elderly patients and those with impaired renal function.

## Conclusion

The effective management of TEN and SJS requires prompt recognition of the conditions, identification and withdrawal of the causative drug, and supportive therapy in an appropriate high-dependency unit, burns unit or intensive care unit. At the present time there is no specific treatment that has been reliably demonstrated to improve the outcome for TEN or SJS.

Current literature relating to the use of IVIg for this indication could be interpreted as encouraging, but results of the larger available studies are conflicting. All are hampered by the lack of control patients, and by the relatively small numbers of cases included (an inevitable problem in this rare condition). Four of the larger studies compare the results of IVIg treatment with historical data on mortality in the literature, and show improved survival.[26,47–49] The one study that attempts to predict mortality for the included cases, based on various measures of severity, shows no benefit from IVIg (but cannot exclude a small benefit).[50] Further interpretation of the available literature is limited by lack of uniformity, both in defining the conditions and in the treatment regimens used, making it difficult to compare studies. Furthermore, the variable rate and extent of progression of both TEN and SJS causes great difficulty in assessing the efficacy of a given intervention in any uncontrolled study. However, the feasibility of organizing a controlled study large enough to detect a significant improvement in outcome from TEN with IVIG has been questioned.[50]

Until further evidence becomes available, the author's personal preference is to use IVIg (in the absence of contraindications) at a dose of 0.75 g/kg/day for 4 days in patients presenting with TEN and SJS, with evidence of extension of epidermal loss over the preceding 24 hours.

# References


1. Lyell A. Toxic epidermal necrolysis: an eruption resembling scalding of the skin. *Br J Dermatol* 1956; **68**: 355–61.

2. Stevens AM, Johnson FC. A new eruptive fever associated with stomatitis and ophthalmia: report of two cases in children. *Am J Dis Child* 1922; **24**: 526–33.

3. Bastuji-Garin S, Rzany B, Stern RS et al. Clinical classification of cases of toxic epidermal necrolysis, Stevens–Johnson syndrome and erythema multiforme. *Arch Dermatol* 1993; **129**: 92–6.

4. Assier H, Bastuji-Garin S, Revuz J et al. Erythema multiforme with mucous membrane involvement and Stevens–Johnson syndrome are clinically different disorders with distinct causes. *Arch Dermatol* 1995; **131**: 539–43.

5. Roujeau JC, Kelly JP, Naldi L et al. Medication use and the risk of Stevens–Johnson syndrome or toxic epidermal necrolysis. *N Engl J Med* 1995; **333**: 1600–7.

6 Saiag P, Caumes E, Chosidow O et al. Drug-induced toxic epidermal necrolysis (Lyell syndrome) in patients infected with the human immunodeficiency virus. *J Am Acad Dermatol* 1992; **26**: 567–74.

7. Villada G, Roujeau J-C, Cordonnier C et al. Toxic epidermal necrolysis after bone marrow transplantation: study of nine cases. *J Am Acad Dermatol* 1990; **23**: 870–5.

8. Wolkenstein P, Revuz J. Toxic epidermal necrolysis. *Dermatol Clin* 2000; **18**: 485–95.

9. Roujeau J-C, Stern RS. Severe adverse cutaneous reactions to drugs. *N Engl J Med* 1994; **331**: 1272–85.

10. Roujeau J-C, Chosidow O, Saiag P et al. Toxic epidermal necrolysis (Lyell syndrome). *J Am Acad Dermatol* 1990; **23**: 1039–58.

11. Shapiro LE, Shear NH. Mechanisms of drug reactions: the metabolic track. *Semin Cutan Med Surg* 1996; **15**: 217–27.

12. Roujeau JC, Huynh TN, Bracq C et al. Genetic susceptibility to toxic epidermal necrolysis. *Arch Dermatol* 1987; **123**: 1171– 3.

13. Wolkenstein P, Carriere V, Charue D et al. A slow acetylator genotype is a risk factor for sulphonamide-induced toxic epidermal necrolysis and Stevens-Johnson syndrome. *Pharmacogenetics* 1995; **5**: 255–8.

14. Friedmann PS, Strickland I, Pirmohamed M et al. Investigation of mechanisms in toxic epidermal necrolysis induced by carbamazepine. *Arch Dermatol* 1994; **130**: 598–604.

15. Wolkenstein P, Charue D, Laurent P et al.

Metabolic predisposition to cutaneous adverse drug reactions. *Arch Dermatol* 1995; **131**: 544–51.

16. Tagami H, Tatsuta K, Iwatski K, Yamada M. Delayed hypersensitivity in ampicillin-induced toxic epidermal necrolysis. *Arch Dermatol* 1983; **119**: 910–13

17. Villada G, Roujeau JC, Clerici T et al. Immunopathology of toxic epidermal necrolysis. *Arch Dermatol* 1992; **128**: 50–3.

18. Miyauchi H, Hosokawa H, Akaeda T et al. T-cell subsets in drug-induced toxic epidermal necrolysis: possible pathogenic mechanism induced by CD8–positive cells. *Arch Dermatol* 1991; **127**: 851–5.

19. Heng MCY, Allen SG. Efficacy of cyclophosphamide in toxic epidermal necrolysis. *J Am Acad Dermatol* 1991; **25**: 778–86.

20. Correia O, Delgado L, Ramos JP et al. Cutaneous T-cell recruitment in toxic epidermal necrolysis. *Arch Dermatol* 1993; **129**: 466–8.

21. Paquet P, Nikkels A, Arrese JE et al. Macrophages and tumour necrosis factor a in toxic epidermal necrolysis. *Arch Dermatol* 1994; **130**: 605–8.

22. Le Cleach L, Roujeau J-C. Toxic epidermal necrolysis. *J Dermatol Treat* 1998; **9**: 35–7.

23. Griffiths CE, Voorhees JJ, Nickoloff BJ. Gamma interferon induces different keratinocyte cellular patterns of expression of HLA-DR and DQ and intercellular adhesion molecule-I (ICAM-I) antigens. *Br J Dermatol* 1989; **120**: 1–8.

24. Paul C, Wolkenstein P, Adle H et al. Apoptosis as a mechanism of keratinocyte death in toxic epidermal necrolysis. *Br J Dermatol* 1996; **134**: 710–14.

25. Wehrli P, Viard I, Bullani R et al. Death receptors in cutaneous biology and disease. *J Invest Dermatol* 2000; **115**: 141–8.

26. Viard I, Wehrli P, Bullani R et al. Inhibition of toxic epidermal necrolysis by blockade of CD95 with human intravenous immunoglobulin. *Science* 1998; **282**: 490–3.

27. Inachi S, Mizutani H, Shimizu M. Epidermal apoptotic cell death in erythema multiforme and Stevens-Johnson syndrome. Contribution of perforin-positive cell infiltration. *Arch Dermatol* 1997; **133**: 845–9.

28. Schnyder B, Frutig K, Mauri-Hellweg D et al. T-cell-mediated cytotoxicity against keratinocytes in sulfamethoxazole-induced skin reaction. *Clin Exp Allergy* 1998; **28**: 1412–17.

29. Garcia-Doval I, LeCleach L, Bocquet H et al. Toxic epidermal necrolysis and Stevens–Johnson syndrome. Does early withdrawal of causative drugs decrease the risk of death? *Arch Dermatol* 2000; **136**: 323–7.

30. Revuz R, Roujeau J-C, Guillaume J-C et al. Treatment of toxic epidermal necrolysis. *Arch Dermatol* 1987; **123**: 1156–8.

31. Craven NM. Management of toxic epidermal necrolysis. *Hosp Med* 2000; **61**: 778–81.

32. Rasmussen JE. Erythema multiforme in children. Response to treatment with systemic corticosteroids. *Br J Dermatol* 1976; **95**: 181–6.

33. Halebian PH, Corder VJ, Madden MR et al. Improved burn center survival of patients with toxic epidermal necrolysis managed without corticosteroids. *Ann Surg* 1986; **205**: 503–12.

34. Guibal F, Bastuji-Garin S, Chosidow O et al. Characteristics of toxic epidermal necrolysis in patients undergoing long-term glucocorticoid therapy. *Arch Dermatol* 1995; **131**: 669–72.

35. Stables GI, Lever RS. Toxic epidermal necrolysis and systemic corticosteroids. *Br J Dermatol* 1993; **128**: 357.

36. Martinez AE, Atherton DJ. High-dose systemic corticosteroids can arrest recurrences of severe mucocutaneous erythema multiforme. *Pediatr Dermatol* 2000; **17**: 87–90.

37. Tripathi A, Ditto AM, Grammer LC et al. Corticosteroid therapy in an additional 13 cases of Stevens–Johnson syndrome: a total series of 67 cases. *Allergy Asthma Proc* 2000; **21**: 101–5.

38. Arévalo JM, Lorente JA, González-Herrada C et al. Treatment of toxic epidermal necrolysis with cyclosporin A. *J Trauma* 2000; **48**: 473–8.

39. Egan CA, Grant WJ, Morris SE et al. Plasmapheresis as an adjunct treatment in toxic epidermal necrolysis. *J Am Acad Dermatol* 1999; **40**: 458–61.

40. Redondo P, Ruiz de Erenchun F, Monedero P et al. Toxic epidermal necrolysis. Treatment with pentoxifylline. *Br J Dermatol* 1994; **130**: 688–9.

41. Redondo P, De Felipe I, De La Pena A et al. Drug induced hypersensitivity syndrome and toxic epidermal necrolysis. Treatment with *N*-acetylcysteine. *Br J Dermatol* 1997; **136**: 645–6.

42. Wolkenstein P, Latarjet J, Roujeau J-C, et al. Randomised comparison of thalidomide versus placebo in toxic epidermal necrolysis. *Lancet* 1998; **352**: 1586–9.

43. Sacher RA. Intravenous immunoglobulin consensus statement. *J Allergy Clin Immunol* 2001; **108**: 139S–46S.

44. Schiavotto C, Ruggeri M, Rodeghiero F. Adverse reactions after high-dose intravenous immunoglobulin: incidence in 83 patients treated for idiopathic thrombocytopenic purpura (ITP) and review of the literature. *Haematologica.* 1993; **78**(6 Suppl 2): 35–40.

45. Rodeghiero F, Castaman G, Vespignani M et al. Erythema multiforme after intravenous immunoglobulin. *Blut* (1998) 56: 145.

46. Amato GM, Travia A, Ziino O. The use of intravenous high-dose immunoglobulins (IGIV) in a case of Stevens–Johnson syndrome. *Pediatr Med Chir* 1992; **14**: 555–6.

47. Morici MV, Galen WK, Shetty AK et al. Intravenous immunoglobulin therapy for children with Stevens–Johnson syndrome. *J Rheumatol* 2000; **27**: 2494–7.

48. Stella M, Cassano P, Bollero D et al. Toxic epidermal necrolysis treated with intravenous high-dose immunoglobulins: our experience. *Dermatology* 2001; **203**: 45–9.

49: Prins C, Kerdel FA, Padilla RS et al. Treatment of toxic epidermal necrolysis with high-dose intravenous immunoglobulin: multicentric retrospective analysis of 48 consecutive cases. *Arch Dermatol* (in press).

50. Bachot N, Revuz J, Roujeau J-C. Intravenous immunoglobulins did not improve mortality and evolution of Stevens–Johnson syndrome or toxic epidermal necrolysis in a prospective non-comparative study. *Arch Dermatol* (in press).

51. Bastuji-Garin S, Fouchard N, Bertocchi M et al. SCORTEN: a severity-of-illness score for toxic epidermal necrolysis. *J Inv Dermatol* 2000; **115**: 149–53.

52. Moudgil A, Porat S, Brunnel P et al. Treatment of Stevens-Johnson syndrome with pooled human intravenous immune globulin. *Clin Pediatr (Phila)* 1995; **34**: 48–51.

53. Sanwo M, Nwadiuko R, Beall G. Use of

intravenous immunoglobulin in the treatment of severe cutaneous drug reactions in patients with AIDS. *J Allergy Clin Immunol* 1996; **98:** 1112–15.

54. Phan TG, Wong RC, Crotty K et al. Toxic epidermal necrolysis in acquired immunodeficiency syndrome treated with intravenous gammaglobulin. *Australas J Dermatol* 1999; **40:** 153–7.

55. Straussberg R, Harel L, Ben-Amitai D et al. Carbamazepine-induced Stevens-Johnson syndrome treated with IV steroids and IVIG. *Pediatr Neurol* 2000; **22:** 231–3.

56. Magina S, Lisboa C, Goncalves E et al. A case of toxic epidermal necrolysis treated with intravenous immunoglobin. *Br J Dermatol* 2000; **142:** 191–2.

57. Eisen ER, Fish J, Shear NH. Management of drug-induced toxic epidermal necrolysis. *J Cutan Med Surg* 2000; **4:** 96–102.

58. Paquet P, Jacob E, Damas P et al. Treatment of drug-induced toxic epidermal necrolysis (Lyell's syndrome) with intravenous human immunoglobulins. *Burns* 2001; **27:** 652–5.

59. Brett AS, Philips D, Lynn AW. Intravenous immunoglobulin therapy for Stevens–Johnson syndrome. *South Med J* 2001; **94:** 342–3.

60. Corne P, Dereure O, Guilhou JJ et al. Toxic epidermal necrolysis treated with intravenous immunoglobulins. *Rev Med Interne* 2001; **22:** 491–2.

# Intravenous immunoglobulin in the treatment of scleromyxoedema, scleroderma, pyoderma gangrenosum and pretibial myxoedema

**7**

Stephen Jolles

CIDP, chronic inflammatory demyelinating polyneuropathy; PG, pyoderma gangrenosum; PUVA, psoralen ultraviolet A; SCIG, subcutaneous immunoglobulin; SSc, systemic sclerosis; TGF-β, transforming growth factor beta; TNF-α, tumour necrosis factor alpha

## Introduction

Intravenous immunoglobulin (IVIg) is a blood product prepared from the serum of between 1000 and 15,000 donors per batch and is the treatment of choice for patients with antibody deficiencies. In these conditions IVIg is used at a 'replacement dose' of 200–400 mg/kg body weight, given approximately 3-weekly. In contrast, 'high-dose' IVIg (hdIVIg), given most frequently at 2 g/kg/month, is used as an 'immunomodulatory' agent in an increasing number of immune and inflammatory disorders. The initial use of hdIVIg was for idiopathic thrombocytopenic purpura (ITP) in children.[1] Despite the lack of double-blind randomized placebo-controlled trials, many other disorders are managed with hdIVIg, including numerous haematological, rheumatological, neurological and dermatological disorders.[2]

For the purposes of clarity IVIg may be considered to have four separate mechanistic components: actions mediated by the variable regions $F(ab')_2$; actions of Fc on a range of Fc receptors (FcR); actions mediated by complement binding within the Fc fragment; and immunomodulatory substances other than antibody in the IVIg preparations. It is likely that these components act concurrently; however, the different mechanisms may vary in importance in different clinical settings. The mechanisms of action have been discussed in Chapter 1 and are summarized here in Table 7.1.[3]

The side-effects of IVIg are generally mild and self-limiting, often occurring 30–60 minutes after the onset of the infusion. They include flushing, myalgia, headache, fever, chills, low backache, nausea or vomiting, chest tightness, wheezing, changes in blood pressure and tachycardia. Aseptic meningitis may occur,[4] and very rarely episodes of anaphylaxis, particularly in those IgA-deficient patients with anti-IgA antibodies. Adverse effects can be

**Table 7.1**
*Immunomodulatory actions of intravenous immunoglobulin*

| Immunomodulatory category | Effects |
|---|---|
| **Effects due to $F(ab')_2$** | Antiproliferative effects<br>Modulation of apoptosis and cell cycle<br>Activation of specific cells<br>Effects on cell adhesion<br>Antibodies to pathogens and superantigens<br>Anti-idiotypes<br>Antibodies to immunoregulatory molecules (cytokines, TCR, CD4, CD5)<br>Effects on cytokine levels |
| **Effects due to Fc receptors** | Inhibition of phagocytosis<br>Inhibition of ADCC<br>Effects on antibody production and recycling<br>Effects on glucocorticoid receptor-binding affinity |
| **Effects due to complement–Fc binding** | Inhibition of deposition of activated complement |
| **Effects due to substances other than Ab within IVIg** | IVIg contains cytokines, cytokine receptors, CD4, MHC class II and stabilizing agents, mainly sugars |

minimized by following the guidelines in the physician's checklist,[2] but are generally easily managed by slowing or stopping the infusion, or by premedication with hydrocortisone, paracetamol and/or antihistamine.[5]

## Physician's checklist prior to high dose IVIg

1. Liver function, renal function, full blood count and hepatitis screen (do not use in rapidly progressive renal disease)
2. Immunoglobulin levels to exclude IgA deficiency. If no IgA present, measure anti-IgA antibodies (see Chapter 9)
3. Exclude high-titre rheumatoid factor and cryoglobulinaemia
4. Preferably ensure that a sufficient supply of a single batch of IVIg is available, to expose the patient to a minimum number of donors
5. Take any baseline specimens, examination findings or photographs required to later document an objective response
6. Follow manufacturer's guidelines regarding reconstitution and rate of infusion (and maintain good hydration and fluid intake)
7. Provide patient information regarding high-dose IVIg therapy and consent
8. Store an aliquot of serum so that any future questions regarding transfusion of infectious agents may be answered (e.g. hepatitis G).

## Scleromyxoedema

Scleromyxoedema is a rare skin disease characterized by the deposition of acid mucopolysaccharides from activated fibroblasts in the dermis. The two main components are a papular skin eruption on the ears, forehead and backs of the hands, and a more generalized woody induration of the skin, which may cause microstomia, reduced mobility and considerable disability (Figs 7.1 and 7.2). The disease is often associated with lymphoproliferative disorders, such as

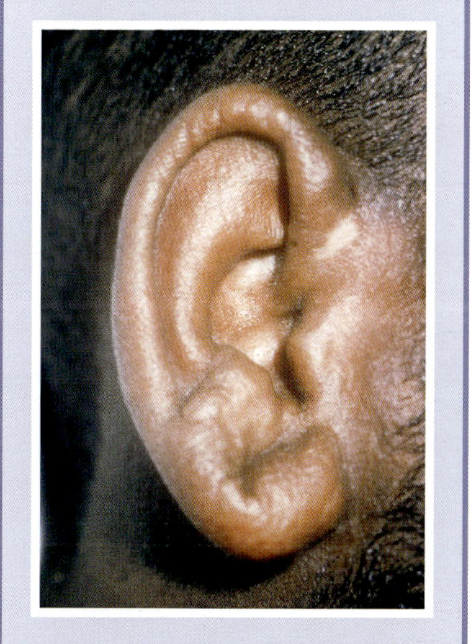

**Fig. 7.1**
*Scleromyxoedema, showing thickened skin.*

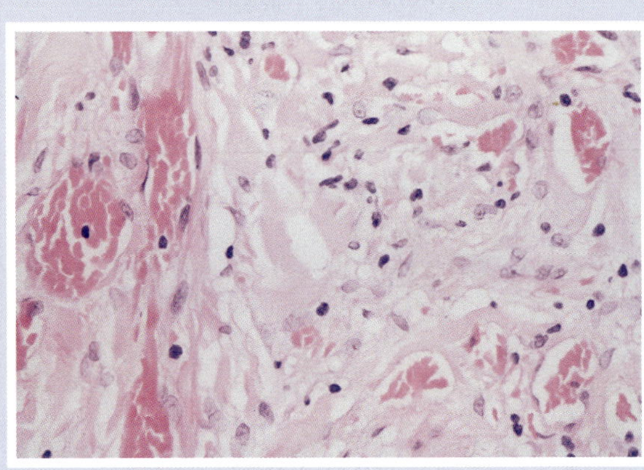

**Fig. 7.2**
*Histology of scleromyxoedema, with the dermal deposition of large amounts of extracellular matrix.*

plasmacytoma, leukaemia and lymphoma. In addition, the majority of patients have an IgG-λ and less commonly an IgG-κ paraprotein.[6,7] A range of extracutaneous manifestations, including polyarthritis, restrictive pulmonary defects, cardiomyopathy, proximal myopathy and oesophageal aperistalsis, have also been described.[6] In view of the rarity of the disorder there have been no randomized controlled studies of treatment and therapeutic data remain largely anecdotal. Reported therapies include cytotoxic agents, PUVA, extracorporeal photopheresis, retinoids, plasmapheresis, interferon-α and cyclosporin.[8]

It is not clear what role the paraprotein plays in the pathogenesis of scleromyxoedema; however, there are precedents for the use of IVIg in conditions with paraproteins. The first is when replacement doses of IVIg are used to prevent infection when a paraprotein is associated with immune paresis and significant hypogammaglobulinaemia (e.g. myeloma); in the second, IVIg is used at high dose in the demyelinating neuropathies, such as chronic inflammatory demyelinating polyneuropathy (CIDP), which may be associated with paraproteins. In CIDP associated with a monoclonal paraprotein the benefit of hdIVIg appeared similar to that in CIPD without a paraprotein, suggesting that the presence of a paraprotein is not necessarily a contraindication to IVIg treatment.[9]

There are five scleromyxoedema patients reported to have been treated with hdIVIg.[8,10] All were given a dose of 2 g/kg/month over 5 days, and improvement was noted in all patients. Two patients reduced their skin scores and three had improvements in both cutaneous and systemic manifestations of their disease. (An additional unpublished case of scleromyxoedema treated with hdIVIg did not respond to this or other treatments; personal communication, Dr Malcolm Rustin.)

One of the most serious aspects of scleromyxoedema is encephalitis, which is associated with a high mortality. It is of particular interest that hdIVIg was observed to improve encephalitis in the two patients with this complication, as perhaps any inflammation involving the blood–brain barrier may have made the CNS more accessible to IVIg. Although the monoclonal antibodies in one patient became undetectable, there were no consistent overall reductions in the level of paraprotein noted. Three of the patients had long-lasting benefit from hdIVIg, allowing the treatment intervals to be increased or IVIg to be withdrawn, and two required ongoing treatment. In view of the lack of understanding of the pathogenesis of scleromyxoedema it is only possible to speculate as to the mechanism of action of hdIVIg in this disorder. It seems likely that serum factor(s) stimulate fibroblasts to divide and produce excessive matrix components, and that IVIg may interfere either with the production or the action of these putative factors. The rarity of this condition makes it difficult to envisage controlled studies being easily carried out, and therefore it will be important to glean as much information as

possible from each subsequent case treated with hdIVIg to allow informed therapeutic decisions to be made.

## Pyoderma gangrenosum

Pyoderma gangrenosum (PG) is a destructive, necrotizing non-infective ulceration of the skin which presents as a furuncle-like nodule, pustule or haemorrhagic bulla (Fig. 7.3). The pathogenesis is not fully understood, and histology reveals sterile abscess formation with venous and capillary thrombosis, haemorrhage, necrosis, and massive cellular infiltration with neutrophils, epithelioid and giant cells. In more chronic forms a more mononuclear cell infiltrate predominates. The advancing border shows features of a lymphocytic vasculitis, suggesting the endothelial cell is an early target.

Differential diagnoses include Behçets

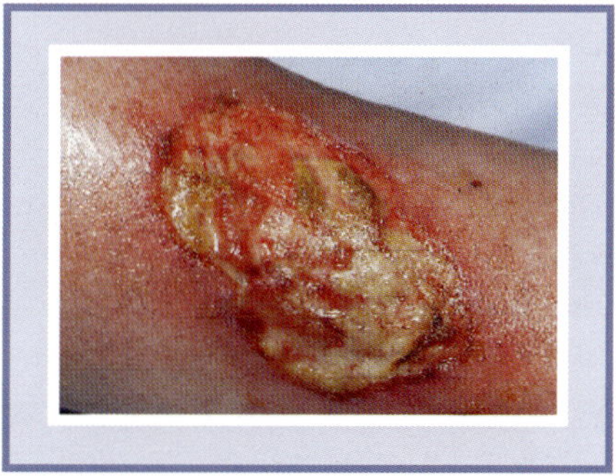

**Fig. 7.3**
*Pyoderma gangrenosum.*

syndrome, other forms of vasculitis (e.g. Wegener's granulomatosis), infections such as microaerophilic streptococcus, *Clostridium welchii*, amoebiasis cutis, cryptococcosis and blastomycosis. PG is associated with conditions involving the gastrointestinal tract (e.g. Crohn's disease), the liver (e.g. chronic active hepatitis), the joints (e.g. rheumatoid arthritis and ankylosing spondylitis) and the blood (e.g. leukaemia and myeloma), as well as other malignancies and trauma. When associated with another underlying disease process, treatment of PG is in the first instance that of the associated disorder. Further treatments include systemic and intralesional steroids, salazopyrin, dapsone, pentoxyphylline in view of its anti-TNF properties, cyclosporin, minocycline and clofazamine.

Three patients have been reported to have been treated with hdIVIg for PG.[11–13] The first was a 35-year-old woman with no identifiable underlying cause for the PG who had received multiple other treatments, including oral, intravenous and intralesional steroids, dapsone and cyclosporin, with no sustained benefit. The ulcer continued to enlarge and hdIVIg was given at 0.4 g/kg/day for 5 days, with improvement within 2 weeks. A second cycle of hdIVIg was given at 1 g/kg/day for 2 days, and sustained benefit was observed in that the ulcer gradually healed and the cyclosporin and prednisolone were reduced. Eight months later the ulcer had not recurred.[11]

The second report describes a 37-year-old woman with large painful PG ulcers on the feet and distal legs for 15 years, who had failed to respond to high-dose oral steroids (prednisolone 80 mg/day) and cyclosporin. The cyclosporin was discontinued because of renal side-effects and hdIVIg (Sandoglobulin 1 g/kg/day for 2 days) introduced as adjunctive therapy with prednisolone at 60 mg/day. Improvement was noted after 1 week and monthly cycles of hdIVIg were continued for 4 months, resulting in complete healing. During this time it was also possible to taper the prednisolone to 10 mg/day.[12] Most recently a 45-year-old female patient with a pre-existing IgGκ monoclonal gammopathy developed post-traumatic PG following a cardiac bypass procedure, and was treated with combination hdIVIg (3 g/kg over 6 days of Polyglobin N) and high-dose steroids, which rapidly halted the progression of the disease.[13]

The three cases reported were all treated adjunctively with hdIVIg and responded rapidly where other therapies had failed. It was also clear that it was possible to reduce other treatments when the lesions had healed, and to discontinue hdIVIg. The mechanism of action is again not clear in this circumstance; however, PG in the setting of hypogammaglobulinaemia has been described to improve with IVIg.[14,15] It is possible that effects of hdIVIg on the local cytokine environment (e.g. levels of TNF-α), particularly at the active edge of the ulcer, where a vasculitic histology is observed, and modification of cellular recruitment into the ulcer may play a role.

## Systemic sclerosis

Systemic sclerosis (SSc) is a multisystem disorder characterized by the association of vascular abnormalities, connective tissue sclerosis and atrophy and autoimmune changes. In the skin it is characterized by fibrosis and obliteration of vessels. It may also occur as a skin-localized form, morphoea.[16]

The pathogenesis of SSc is not fully understood, but examination of tissues from patients indicates that early disease is characterized by the activation of endothelial cells and fibroblasts and by tissue infiltration with activated lymphocytes (predominantly T cells), especially in perivascular areas.[17,18] E-selectin is increased on SSc endothelial cells, and this may facilitate lymphocyte homing to skin. A number of growth factors, including interleukin-1 (IL-1) and transforming growth factor-β (TGF-β) have been implicated in stimulating fibroblast production of collagen and other matrix components such as glycoaminoglycans, leading to tissue fibrosis. Disease progression is associated with endothelial cell damage and loss, intimal proliferation, luminal narrowing and thrombosis, and fibrosis of small arteries and capillaries. Late in the disease, mononuclear cell infiltration may resolve and fibrosis may lessen.

There are four reported patients with SSc who have been treated with hdIVIg.[19,20] In a preliminary study of the efficacy of this treatment in SSc two women aged 20 and 28 years and a man aged 48 years with diffuse cutaneous sclerosis were given hdIVIg as monotherapy.[19] They had previously all been treated with colchicine, and the man had also received D-penicillamine without benefit. The PM-Scl autoantibody titre was measured by immunofluorescence before and after the treatment, and before and after each cycle of hdIVIg. All three patients had major reductions in skin scores (modified Rodnan total skin thickness score) occurring between the second and third cycles of treatment. Both women completed six cycles of 2 g/kg/month of hdIVIg and skin scores remained stable 3 years later. The male patient, however, developed hypertension 3 weeks following the third hdIVIg infusion, and over the next 3 weeks progressed into renal failure and died of sepsis. The authors conclude that it cannot be ruled out that hdIVIg was the cause of his renal failure, but that this was unlikely. SSc carries a risk of renal crisis, particularly in the first year of disease; in addition, high-titre rheumatoid factor may be associated with immune complex-mediated renal failure following hdIVIg.[5]

The fourth patient suffered from a long-standing SSc/DM (dermatomyositis) overlap

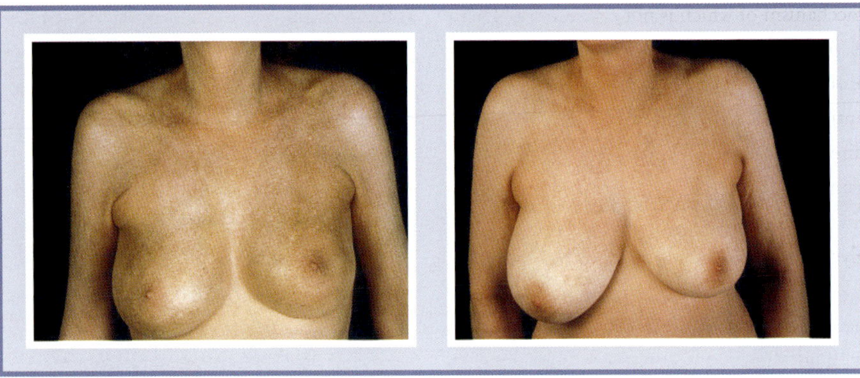

**Fig. 7.4**
*Patient pre- and post-hdIVIg for scleroderma, note the changes in both skin pigmentation stiffness (with kind permission from Professor T Luger).*

syndrome.[20] She had generalized fibrosis, myositis, skin hyperpigmentation, sclerodactyly, Raynaud's phenomenon and oesophageal sclerosis (Fig. 7.4). She was treated with 10 cycles of adjunctive hdIVIg (2 g/kg/month) with low-dose prednisolone. The muscle weakness improved after 4 months, and after 10 months the skin thickening and oesophageal dysfunction had also improved markedly, allowing a gradual reduction in prednisolone over a 6-month period without disease relapse.

A further report describes an 11-year-old boy with disabling pansclerotic morphoea of childhood who was treated with hdIVIg (1.2g/kg of Alphaglobin) at variable intervals, but most effectively when given monthly.[21] This resulted in the healing of extensive lower limb ulcers, and the authors suggest that this may have been due to the antibacterial effects of IVIg. This may be part of the explanation, but the boy did not have a documented humoral immunodeficiency and was treated with three times the replacement dose of IVIg which may have had other disease-modifying effects.

## Pretibial myxoedema

These are localized oedematous and thickened pretibial plaques which develop rarely in patients with hyperthyroidism due to Graves' disease. Three clinical types are recognized: nodular, diffuse and elephantiasic. Histology reveals an excessive dermal and subcutaneous deposition of glycosaminoglycans, the mechanism of which is not understood. There is, however, some *in vitro* evidence that antithyroid-stimulating hormone receptor antibodies (anti-TSH receptor) may be directed against thyroid antigens on pretibial skin fibroblasts and adipocytes, stimulating them to secrete large amounts of glycosaminoglycans.[22,23]

There are two reports totalling eight patients with pretibial myxoedema treated with hdIVIg.[24,25] In the first, seven patients with Graves' ophthalmopathy and pretibial myxoedema (four with nodular, two with diffuse, and one with elephantiasic types) were treated with hdIVIg.[24] Endobulin Immuno was given to six patients at 2 g/kg over 5 days every 3 weeks; the same dose was then subsequently given over 1 day for between 7 and 15 cycles. The remaining patient with elephantiasic pretibial myxoedema was given Veinoglobuline (Institut Mérieux, Lyon, France) using the same protocol. Clinical improvement of pretibial myxoedema and Graves' ophthalmopathy was noted in all patients (in four the lesions disappeared), with a reduction of pretibial skin thickness on ultrasonography. Four patients had a reduction in the mucopolysaccharide level in the skin, in three lymphocytic skin infiltration disappeared, and in two IgG deposition decreased. A parallel reduction in the titre of circulating autoantibodies (antithyroglobulin, antimicrosomal, anti-TSH receptor, antinuclear, antismooth muscle, and antimitochondrial) was observed. Two control patients with Graves' ophthalmopathy and pretibial myxoedema treated with systemic corticosteroids did not show any improvement in the skin.

The second report describes a disease-stabilizing effect of hdIVIg (2 g/kg/month for six cycles) in a 36-year-old women with long-standing elephantiasic pretibial myxoedema.[25] There was no major change in the levels of hexuronic acid in the skin 1 month after treatment, and a 50% reduction in anti-TSH receptor antibodies was achieved after five cycles. At 1-year follow-up the anti-TSH receptor antibody titre had returned to slightly higher than pretreatment levels, without disease progression. The authors suggest that this reduction may have been insufficient to have a greater effect on the disease process, and that long-standing elephantiasic pretibial myxoedema remains a therapeutic challenge.

## Psoriasis

A recent study into the use of adjunctive hdIVIg in three female patients with psoriasis describes rapid improvement in the rheumatological aspects of their disease with reductions in inflammatory markers in all patients.[26] The psoriatic skin changes improved dramatically in two and became less severe in one though involved the same area of skin. Skin responses were rapid in one and more gradual in the remainder. The authors

**Table 7.2**
Summary of scleromyxoedema, pyoderma gangrenosum, scleroderma and pretibial myxoedema reports

| Disease | No. of Patients | Demographics | Dose & frequency | Preparation | Additional treatment | Outcome | Response time | Duration | Reference |
|---|---|---|---|---|---|---|---|---|---|
| Scleromyxoedema | 5 | 2F 3M 30–74 yrs | 2 g/kg/month given over 5 days | Octagam in 2, Sandoglobulin in 3 | Prednisolone in 1 Monotherapy in 4 | Improved in all but relapse in 1 | 2 weeks to 6 month for full response | Weeks to months | Lister,[10] Righi,[8] |
| Pyoderma gangrenosum | 3 | 3F 35–45 yrs | 2 g/kg/month given over 2–5 days in 2 and 3 g/kg over 6 days in 1 | Sandoglobulin in 1, Polyglobin N in 1, N/A in 1 | All adjunctive, Prednisolone in 2, Prednisolone and cyclosporin in 1 | Improved in all | 1–2 weeks | Weeks to months, allowing reduction in other therapies | Gupta[11] Dirschka[12] Gleichmann[13] |
| Scleroderma | 4 | 3F 1M 28–49 yrs | 2 g/kg/month | ISIVEN in 3 and N/A in 1 | Monotherapy in 3 Adjunctive in 1 | Improved in all (one patient died 6 wks after third cycle of hdIVIg) | 2–4 months | May be long-lasting when in remission after 6–10 cycles of hdIVIg | Rutter[20] Levy[19] |
| Pretibial myxoedema | 8 | 5F 3M 36–67 yrs | 2 g/kg/month in 1, 2 g/kg/ 3 weeks in 7 | Endobulin in 6 Veinoglobulin in 1 and N/A in 1 | Monotherapy in all | 7 improved 1 disease progression halted | 2–9 months | Long-lasting when in remission | Antonelli[24] Terheyden[25] |

speculate that the mechanism may involve effects on TNF-α, as inhibitors of this cytokine have been shown to have efficacy in the treatment of psoriasis.

## Discussion

The conditions described are linked by the fact that scleromyxoedema, scleroderma and pretibial myxoedema are associated with skin thickening due to the production of either excessive collagen or glycosaminoglycans or other matrix components, whereas in scleroderma and pyoderma gangrenosum endothelial cell injury appears to be critical.

The evidence base for hdIVIg in all these disorders is small and consists of case reports and small case series (summarized in Table 7.2). The reports are likely to reflect a bias for positive results, and it is therefore difficult to draw firm conclusions. It is also not possible to be certain about the mechanism of action of hdIVIg, as in most cases the pathogenesis of the disease itself is not understood. However, there does appear to be either a direct or an indirect effect of hdIVIg on skin extracellular matrix turnover. This turnover is dependent on the rate at which matrix is laid down versus its removal, which is likely to be influenced by a number of cell types, including endothelial cells, fibroblasts and, potentially, lymphocytes and their respective activation states. The known mechanisms of action of hdIVIg (summarized in Table 7.1) which may influence matrix turnover are either local, such as alteration of the cytokine milieu, effects on cellular migration by blocking adhesion events; or systemic, such as modulation of autoantibody levels (anti-TSH receptor) or other circulating factors. It is also possible that the generation of excess matrix components may allow the binding of cytokines and chemokines, protecting them from breakdown and maintaining an enhanced gradient facilitating both cellular migration into and activation/proliferation of cells within the skin.

It would certainly be of interest to study whether the local administration of subcutaneous immunoglobulin (SCIg) delivering a high dose to the disease site (e.g. in pyoderma gangrenosum) would be effective compared with hdIVIg.

There is much to learn about the mechanism of action of hdIVIg in these conditions, and the challenge will be to design appropriately controlled trials to determine whether the encouraging initial results are maintained. In the majority of cases the effect of hdIVIg was long-lasting once the disease was in remission and the withdrawal of hdIVIg and other agents was possible. This has implications for both trial design and the potential requirements for this scarce resource.

## Acknowledgements

I would like to thank Dr Jenny Hughes for careful reading of the manuscript. Stephen

Jolles is supported by the Leukaemia Research Foundation and the Peel Medical Research Trust.

# References

1.   Imbach P, Barandun S, d'Apuzzo V et al. High-dose intravenous gammaglobulin for idiopathic thrombocytopenic purpura in childhood. *Lancet* 1981; **i**: 1228–31.

2.   Jolles S, Hughes J, Whittaker S. Dermatological uses of high-dose intravenous immunoglobulin. *Arch Dermatol* 1998; **134**: 80–6.

3.   Sewell WAC, Jolles S. Immunomodulatory action of intravenous immunoglobulin (IVIG). *Immunology* 2002; (in press).

4.   Jolles S, Hill H. Management of aseptic meningitis secondary to intravenous immunoglobulin. *Br Med J* 1998; **316**: 936.

5.   Misbah SA, Chapel HM. Adverse effects of intravenous immunoglobulin. *Drug Safety* 1993; **9**: 254–62.

6.   Dinneen AM, Dicken CH. Scleromyxedema. *J Am Acad Dermatol* 1995; **33**: 37–43.

7.   Lai a Fat RF, Suurmond D, Radl J, van Furth R. Scleromyxoedema (lichen myxoedematosus) associated with a paraprotein, IgG 1 of type kappa. *Br J Dermatol* 1973; **88**: 107–16.

8.   Righi A, Schiavon F, Jablonska S et al. Intravenous immunoglobulins control scleromyxoedema. *Ann Rheum Dis* 2002; **61**: 59–61.

9.   van Doorn PA. Chronic inflammatory demyelinating polyneuropathy. In: Said G, ed. *Treatment of Neurological Disorders with Intravenous Immunoglobulins.* London: Martin Dunitz, 44–56.

10.  Lister RK, Jolles S, Whittaker S et al. Scleromyxedema: response to high-dose intravenous immunoglobulin (hdIVIg). *J Am Acad Dermatol* 2000; **43**: 403–8.

11.  Gupta AK, Shear NH, Sauder DN. Efficacy of human intravenous immune globulin in pyoderma gangrenosum. *J Am Acad Dermatol* 1995; **32**: 140–2.

12.  Dirschka T, Kastner U, Behrens S, Altmeyer P. Successful treatment of pyoderma gangrenosum with intravenous human immunoglobulin. *J Am Acad Dermatol* 1998; **39**: 789–90.

13.  Gleichmann US, Otte HG, Korfer R, Stadler R. [Post-traumatic pyoderma gangrenosum: combination therapy with intravenous immunoglobulins and systemic corticosteroids]. *Hautarzt* 1999; **50**: 879–83.

14.  Marcussen PV. Hypogammaglobulinemia in pyoderma gangrenosum. *J Invest Dermatol* 1955; **24**: 275–80.

15.  Bloom D, Fisher D, Dannenberg M. Pyoderma gangrenosum associated with hypogammaglobulinemia. *Arch Dermatol* 1958; **77**: 412–21.

16.  Rowell NR, Goodfield MJD. The connective tissue diseases. In: Champion RH, Burton JL, Burns DA, Breathnach SM eds, 6th Edn, Vol. 3, Oxford: Blackwell Science, *Textbook of Dermatology* 1998; 2437–575

17.  Sollberg S, Peltonen J, Uitto J, Jimenez SA. Elevated expression of beta 1 and beta 2 integrins, intercellular adhesion molecule 1, and endothelial leukocyte adhesion molecule 1 in the skin of patients with systemic sclerosis of recent onset. *Arthritis Rheum* 1992; **35**: 290–8.

18. Prescott RJ, Freemont AJ, Jones CJ, Hoyland J, Fielding P. Sequential dermal microvascular and perivascular changes in the development of scleroderma. *J Pathol* 1992; **166**: 255–63.

19. Levy Y, Sherer Y, Langevitz P et al. Skin score decrease in systemic sclerosis patients treated with intravenous immunoglobulin – a preliminary report. *Clin Rheumatol* 2000; **19**: 207–11.

20. Rutter A, Luger TA. High-dose intravenous immunoglobulins: an approach to treat severe immune-mediated and autoimmune diseases of the skin. *J Am Acad Dermatol* 2001; **44**: 1010–24.

21. Wollina U, Looks A, Schneider R, Maak B. Disabling morphoea of childhood-beneficial effect of intravenous immunoglobulin therapy. *Clin Exp Dermatol* 1998; **23**, 292–3.

22. Chang TC, Wu SL, Hsiao YL et al. TSH and TSH receptor antibody-binding sites in fibroblasts of pretibial myxedema are related to the extracellular domain of entire TSH

receptor. *Clin Immunol Immunopathol* 1994; **71**: 113–20.

23. Young DA, Evans CH, Smith TJ. Leukoregulin induction of protein expression in human orbital fibroblasts: evidence for anatomical site-restricted cytokine-target cell interactions. *Proc Natl Acad Sci USA* 1998; **95**: 8904–9.

24. Antonelli A, Navarranne A, Palla R et al. Pretibial myxedema and high-dose intravenous immunoglobulin treatment. *Thyroid* 1994; **4**: 399–408.

25. Terheyden P, Kahaly G, Zillikens D, Broeker E-B. Treatment of elephantiasic pretibial myxedema with high dose intravenous immunoglobulin. *Br J Dermatol* 2002; (in press).

26. Gurmin V, Rustin MH, Beynon HL. (2002) Psoriasis: response to high-dose intravenous immunoglobulin in three patients. *Br J Dermatol,* **147**: 554–7.

# IVIg therapy in autoimmune mucocutaneous blistering diseases

## A Razzaque Ahmed and Naveed Sami

BP, bullous pemphigoid; CP, cicatricial pemphigoid; EBA, epidermolysis bullosa acquisita; HG, herpes gestationis; LABD, linear IgA bullous disease; OP, oral pemphigoid; PF, pemphigus foliaceus; PV, pemphigus vulgaris

## Introduction

Autoimmune mucocutaneous blistering diseases are a group of rare dermatological diseases,[1] Their exact incidence is not known, as patients are treated by multiple specialists and laws do not mandate the reporting of these diseases to state healthcare authorities. In many patients the diagnosis is missed, leading to potentially irreversible complications and/or death.

In the past, the mortality in many of these diseases was exceedingly high, often due to secondary complications.[2] Since the discovery of systemic corticosteroid therapy, high-dose systemic corticosteroids have been shown to be successful in controlling such diseases.[3] A significant number of serious sides-effects, which required medical intervention, were reported from the long-term usage of high-dose systemic corticosteroid therapy.[4] Some patients died as a consequence of these complications.

In the 1970s, a group of immunosuppressive agents (ISA) were used as adjunctive therapy with systemic corticosteroids, for their steroid-sparing effects.[5] These drugs had been used earlier in organ transplant patients.[6] As new immunosuppressive agents were discovered, they were used in patients with severe disease. Some of these include azathioprine, methotrexate, gold, cyclophosphamide, cylosporin and mycophenolate mofetil.[1–7] The purpose of using these agents is to inhibit the production of pathogenic autoantibodies.

However, these ISA have severe short- and long-term side effects from prolonged immune suppression, frequently resulting in the discontinuation of their use.[8] Some of them have been recently associated with enhanced predisposition to the development of certain cancers, as a result of long-term usage.[9] In such patients, alternative treatment modalities have been used.

Intravenous immunoglobulin (IVIg) is a biological agent that has been used to treat various autoimmune diseases and chronic inflammatory diseases.[10] In this chapter we will discuss the indications, the protocols used and outcome measures in the management of various autoimmune mucocutaneous blistering diseases, including pemphigus vulgaris, pemphigus foliaceus, cicatricial pemphigoid, bullous pemphigoid, linear IgA bullous disease, epidermolysis bullosa acquisita and herpes gestationis.

# Pemphigus vulgaris

Pemphigus vulgaris (PV) is an autoimmune blistering disease which can affect both the skin and the mucous membranes of the oral cavity, nose, eye, pharynx, larynx, esophagus, anal canal, penis and vagina.[1] The majority of patients have a mean age of onset of 50–60 years, and the disease affects both genders equally. The exact incidence of the disease is not known. However, various studies in different areas of the world have reported it to be between 0.42 and 0.5 cases per 100,000. In the Jewish population the incidence is reported to be 1.62–3.2 per 100,000.[1] On indirect immunofluorescence, the presence in the sera of patients of antibodies to the intercellular cement substance (ICS), or keratinocyte cell surface, is considered typical of PV[11] (Fig. 8.1). Recently developed newer technologies can detect the presence of more specific autoantibodies in PV. Patients with mucosal involvement have been recently described to have autoantibodies to desmoglein 3.[12] The presence of autoantibody to desmoglein 1 has been observed in patients with PV who also have cutaneous lesions.[12]

Systemic corticosteroids and

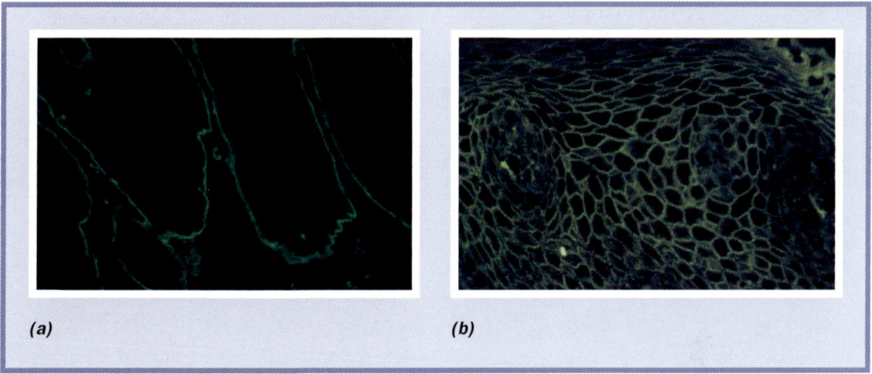

**Fig. 8.1**
*(a) Monkey esophagus substrate reacted with serum from a patient with BP. Note a smooth homogenous binding on the basement membrane zone (BMZ). (b) Monkey esophagus reacted with serum from a patient with PV. Note binding to the ICS.*

immunosuppressive agents have been conventionally used to treat PV.[1] However, despite therapeutically effective doses of various combinations of immunosuppressive agents, the mortality rate among PV patients remains at 10–15%.[13]

The first use of IVIg therapy in PV was reported in 1989.[14] Its use has been described in 57 patients who continue to have severe progressive disease, often unresponsive to conventional therapy[14–24] (Table 8.1). One study has described the use of IVIg in a unique subset of pemphigus patients who had serologic features of both PF and PV.[25]

In the initial studies in the English literature there were 21 patients with PV who were treated with IVIg therapy.[14–22] However, there were many shortcomings in these studies which allowed only limited conclusions to be drawn about the role of IVIg therapy. The administration of IVIg therapy, along with concurrent treatments, and follow-up varied in these reports. The patients received IVIg at a dose of 1–2 g/kg per cycle, administered over a period of 3–5 days, which was defined as one cycle. Eight of the 21 patients received only one cycle. Thirteen patients received multiple cycles. The frequency of cycles and the duration of treatment varied. These parameters were often determined by the observed clinical response. In eight of the 13 patients who received multiple cycles, IVIg was administered at a frequency intervals ranging from every 2 to 4 weeks. In the five remaining patients who

**Table 8.1**
*Clinical data on IVIg therapy in autoimmune mucocutaneous blistering diseases*

| Disease | Total no. of patients | Ages (yrs) | Gender | IVIg dose | * Initial frequency of IVIg cycles | Duration to achieve effective clinical response | Clinical outcome |
|---|---|---|---|---|---|---|---|
| Pemphigus vulgaris[14–24] | 57 | 27–80 | 27 M 30 F | 250–400 mg/ kg/day × 3–5 days | 2–4-week intervals | Days to 6.5 months | Remission (52 patients) |
| Pemphigus foliaceus[17,25,28-30] | 28 | 27–79 | 12 M 16 F | 40–400 mg/kg/ day × 3–5 days | 3–4-week intervals | 3 wks to 6 months | Remission (26 patients) Clinical control (2 patients) |
| Cicatricial pemphigoid[40-45] | 43 | 36–77 | 26 F 17 M | 350–1000 mg/ kg/day × 2–3 days | 2–4-week intervals | 2.7–6.4 months | Remission (41 patients) Clinical control (2 patients) |
| Bullous pemphigoid[14,17,21,33,35] | 34 | 61–89 | 20 M 14 F | 100–400 mg/kg/ day × 3–5 days | 4-week intervals | 2–4 months | Remission (20 patients) |
| Epidermolysis bullosa acquisita[21,47-54] | 8 | 16–63 | 8 M | 40 mg–2 g/kg/day × 3–5 days | 2–4-week intervals | 3–4 months | Clinical control (8 patients) |
| Linear IgA bullous disease[59-61] | 3 | 50–67 | 2 M 1 F | 1–2 g/kg/cycle × 3–4 days | 2–4-week intervals | 4.5 months | Remission (2 patients) Clinical control (1 patient) |
| Herpes gestationis[63] | 1 | 17 | 1 F | 400 mg/kg/day × 5 days | 5 weeks | NA | Clinical control |

*In references 23–25, 28, 29, 35, 40–45, 54, 59, 61 and 63 the intervals of IVIg therapy were gradually prolonged once effective clinical control was achieved to every 6, 8, 10, 12, 14 and 16 weeks.
NA, Not available.

were observed to have a clinical response after the first cycle, IVIg was given when patients developed acute exacerbations and recurrences.

Seventeen of the 21 patients were reported to have improvement after multiple doses of IVIg therapy. In three of the four patients who were reported as having failed to respond to IVIg therapy, only a single dose had been administered. Hence, it would appear that multiple infusions were needed, over a prolonged period of time, to provide clinical benefit.

Recent studies have reported the use of a uniform protocol for IVIg therapy in PV.

These studies used a dose of IVIg a similar to that previously reported, of 1–2 g/kg per cycle.[23,24] This was initially administered every 4 weeks, until an effective clinical response was observed. Effective clinical response was defined as the time at which all previous lesions had healed and no new lesions were observed. This was reported to be a mean of 4.5 months (Figs 8.2 and 8.3). Thereafter, the IVIg was gradually 'tapered'. The concept of tapering IVIg in the treatment of autoimmune blistering diseases is similar to that used with systemic corticosteroids and immunosuppressive agents. Similarly, once a sustained clinical response was observed, the frequency of intervals between IVIg cycles was increased to every 6, 8, 10, 12, 14 and 16 weeks.

Another key issue observed in earlier studies is that patients continued to receive their previous conventional treatments during and/or after receiving IVIg therapy. Hence, IVIg was used as adjunctive therapy with systemic corticosteroids and immunosuppressive agents. This made it difficult to isolate the influence of IVIg on the clinical course of the disease.

However, later studies have demonstrated that once IVIg therapy is instituted, all previous immunosuppressive agents have been discontinued. Hence, IVIg can then be used as monotherapy. In patients whose disease was steroid dependent, IVIg therapy has also been used to provide a steroid-sparing effect.[24] This has also been demonstrated in patients in whom immunosuppressive therapy was contraindicated and who were treated only with systemic prednisone. The difference between the doses of systemic corticosteroids pre- and post-IVIg therapy have been observed to be statistically significant.[23,24] This is particularly important as it has allowed the reduction of both short- and long-term side-effects and medical complications, which can often result in hospitalization. The number of side-effects and days of hospitalization were directly related to the total amount of systemic corticosteroids received.[23]

IVIg monotherapy may be a potential therapeutic option. When IVIg is used with adjunctive therapy, it is difficult to determine which agents actually produced the clinical effect. Moreover, IVIg is used when conventional therapy has failed. It is not clear whether there is any benefit in continuing adjunctive therapy when it has been ineffective.

An important feature of these two large single-center studies is that there was a defined endpoint to the IVIg therapy. Endpoint was defined as the continued absence of disease between two infusion cycles 16 weeks apart. The total number of cycles received by each patient varied according to the severity of their initial disease and their response during the course of treatment. The mean number of cycles that patients received was 18 over a

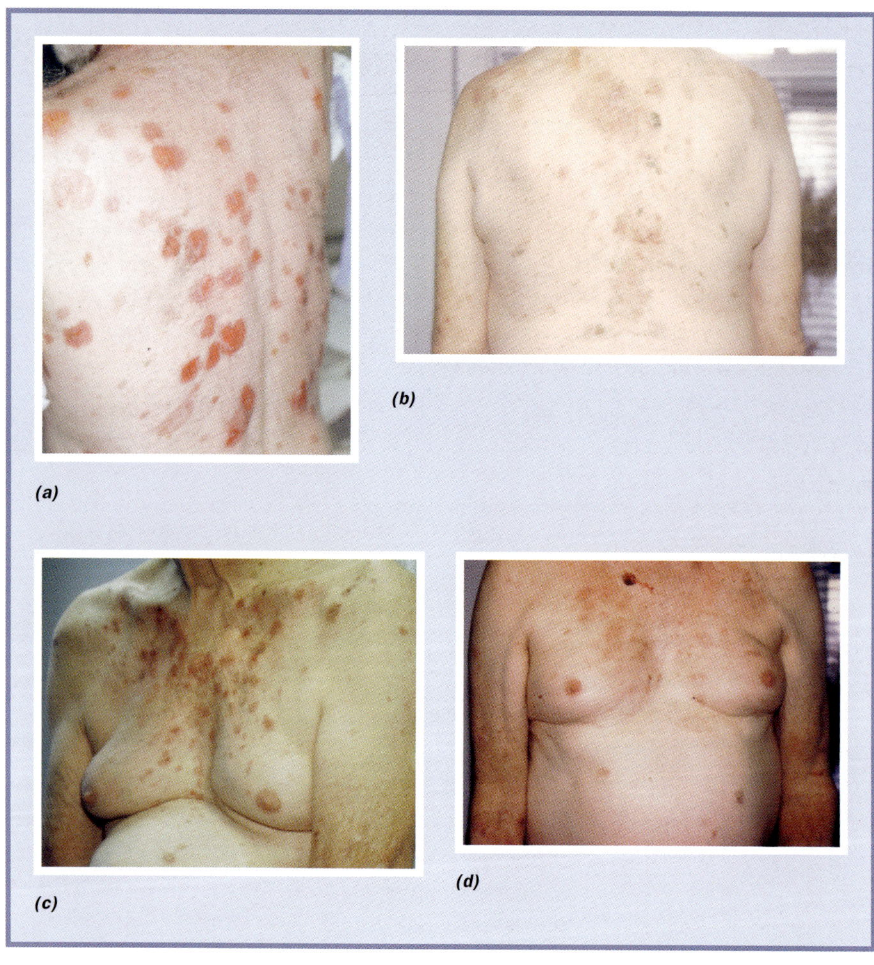

**Fig. 8.2**
*Pemphigus vulgaris pre- and post- IVIg therapy. (a) Multilple widespread lesions of pemphigus vulgaris present on the back pre-IVIg therapy. (b) In the same patient, note complete healing of the lesions on the back post-IVIg therapy. (c) Multiple lesions of pemphigus vulgaris on the chest pre-IVIg therapy. (d) In the same patient, note complete healing of the lesions on the chest post-IVIg therapy.*

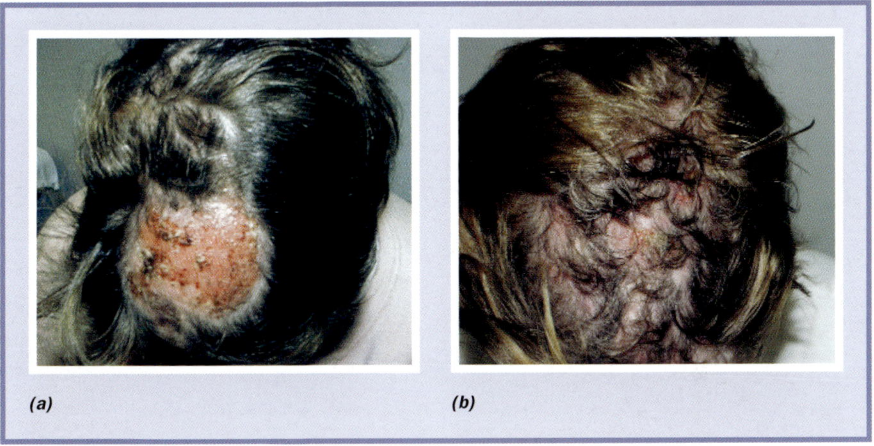



**Fig. 8.3**
*Pemphigus vulgaris pre- and post- IVIg therapy (a) Pemphigus vulgaris lesions involving the scalp and resulting in alopecia pre-IVIg therapy. (b) Note healing of the lesion on the scalp and subsequent significant hair growth post-IVIg therapy.*

mean period of 27 months. Once a clinical remission was induced by IVIg therapy, these patients remained in sustained remission for a relatively long-term follow-up period of observation.

## Pemphigus foliaceus

Pemphigus foliaceus (PF) is an autoimmune blistering disease which primarily affects the skin. It is further subdivided into endemic and non-endemic forms.[1] PF is considered to be more benign than PV. However, some patients may progress to a severe clinical phenotype with exfoliative erythroderma.[1] The pathogenesis of PF is mediated by an autoantibody that targets desmoglein 1, a 160 kDa epidermal protein.[12] Patients with PF require treatment with systemic corticosteroids and immunosuppressive agents.[1] However, there are numerous reports describing PF patients who are unresponsive to conventional therapy and require newer treatment modalities.[26,27] The use of IVIg therapy has been described in only non-endemic PF.[17,25,28–30]

The number of PF patients who have been reported to be treated with IVIg is smaller than those with PV, primarily because PV is more common than PF. There are a total of four studies in the English literature that have described the use of IVIg in patients with PF

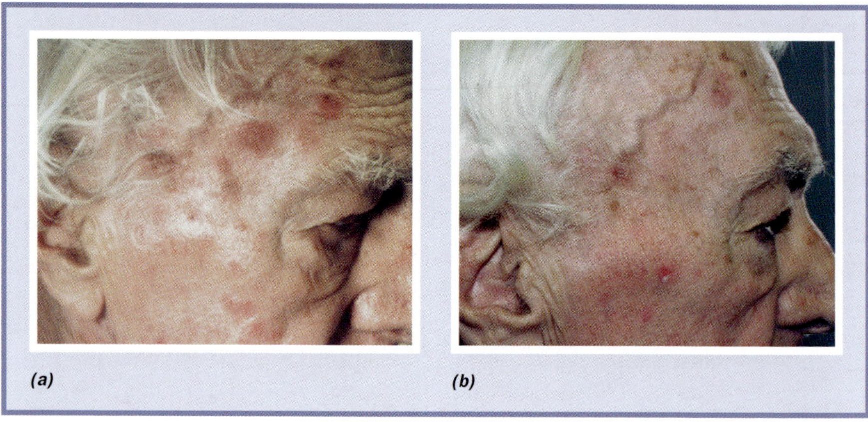

**Fig. 8.4**
*Pemphigus foliaceus pre- and post- IVIg therapy (a) Multiple lesions of pemphigus foliaceus present on the face pre-IVIg therapy. (b) In the same patient, note complete healing of the lesions on the face post-IVIg therapy.*

only.[17,28–30] One study has described the use of IVIg in a unique subset of pemphigus patients who had serological features of both PF and PV.[25]

Because many practicing dermatologists consider PF to be benign, or less severe than PV, the appropriate time to use IVIg may be delayed. In PF, in certain clinical situations the use of IVIg may be considered clinically indicated. These include (1) severe disease, which can be empirically defined when more than 30% of body surface area is involved; (2) failure of multiple systemic agents to induce a prolonged clinical remission; (3) systemic corticosteroid dependence; and (4) contraindications to the use of conventional systemic agents.[17,25,28–30]

The doses described in the literature which have proved effective have ranged between 1 and 2 g/kg per cycle.[25,28,29] However, the successful use of lower doses of IVIg has also been reported.[17,30] These cycles have been administered at initial intervals of every 4 weeks until an effective clinical response is seen, similar to patients with PV. This response is generally attained after a mean of 5–6 months after the initiation of IVIg therapy (Fig. 8.4). Both systemic corticosteroids and other systemic adjuvant agents are gradually tapered and eventually discontinued. The difference in the total doses and durations of systemic corticosteroids pre- and post-IVIg therapy has been shown to be statistically significant. This would suggest that IVIg can also be used as a steroid-sparing agent in PF.[29]

An interesting observation is that patients receiving a higher dosage of IVIg have been observed to have a quicker response than those receiving lower doses. These patients have also been able to discontinue systemic corticosteroids much earlier than those receiving lower doses of IVIg.[17,25,28,29]

Once an effective clinical response has been established, the frequency of intervals between cycles is prolonged to every 6, 8, 10, 12, 14 and 16 weeks.[25,28,29] When patients have no new lesions 16-weeks after the last infusion they are considered to be in remission, and this has been described as the endpoint of therapy. All 26 patients who have followed this protocol have continued in a sustained clinical remission over a long-term follow-up. In one study, IVIg therapy was stopped abruptly once an effective clinical response was observed. However, this patient continued to receive lower doses of systemic prednisone. Because long-term follow-up was not available, the final clinical outcome cannot be evaluated.

## Bullous pemphigoid

Bullous pemphigoid (BP) is a subepidermal bullous skin disease that affects both genders equally. Patients present with tense blisters which are primarily localized to the skin, often in an acral distribution. Indirect immunofluorescence studies using monkey esophagus as substrate detect the presence of anti-BMZ antibody in the sera of patients with BP (Fig. 8.1).[11] The presence of autoantibodies to basement membrane BP Ag 1 and BP Ag 2 in the sera of patients is considered specific and characteristic of BP.[31,32] Conventional therapy includes the use of systemic corticosteroids, anti-inflammatory drugs and immunosuppressive agents. Because BP primarily affects an older age group, the clinical course of the disease and its treatment choices can be influenced by other factors, such as additional medical problems, e.g. diabetes, anemia, cancers, and their treatments. In a subset of patients unresponsive to the conventional agents available to control the disease, IVIg therapy has proved to be a valuable addition to the management of BP.

The use of IVIg in treating BP and nodular pemphigoid has been described in five studies with a total of 34 patients.[14,17,21,33–35] In 33 patients the pemphigoid could not be controlled with systemic corticosteroids and multiple immunosuppressive agents. IVIg therapy was therefore given at a dose of 2 g/kg per cycle.[35] Patients who did not respond had received either a lower dose or only one cycle.[21,33] These patients required higher doses of systemic corticosteroids as well as other treatment modalities, such as plasmapharesis.[33]

Such patients are at a risk of developing

significant complications from these medications, such as steroid-induced diabetes mellitus, osteoporosis, peptic ulcer disease, worsening hypertension and opportunistic infections,[35] often requiring hospitalization. The number of days for hospitalization has been observed to correlate with the total dose of prednisone used. These complications can further retard the healing process. One of the main objectives of using IVIg therapy is to discontinue these conventional treatments as soon as possible, to avoid these side-effects and to facilitate the healing process.

It has been observed in our preliminary studies, and in previous studies, that patients who fail to respond to multiple conventional agents and are corticosteroid dependent, may require multiple cycles to control their disease.[17,21,34,35] It has also been observed that IVIg is most effective when used according to the defined protocol of infusions, initially every 4 weeks. When patients receive multiple cycles, an effective clinical response can be observed over a mean period of 3 months (Fig. 8.5). In some patients clinical improvement may be seen earlier. This control can be maintained as the intervals between infusions cycles is prolonged. The effectiveness of IVIg therapy has also been documented with a statistically significant reduction in the number of relapses and recurrences pre- and post-IVIg therapy.

It is preferable to use IVIg as monotherapy in BP. This is because if multiple agents are

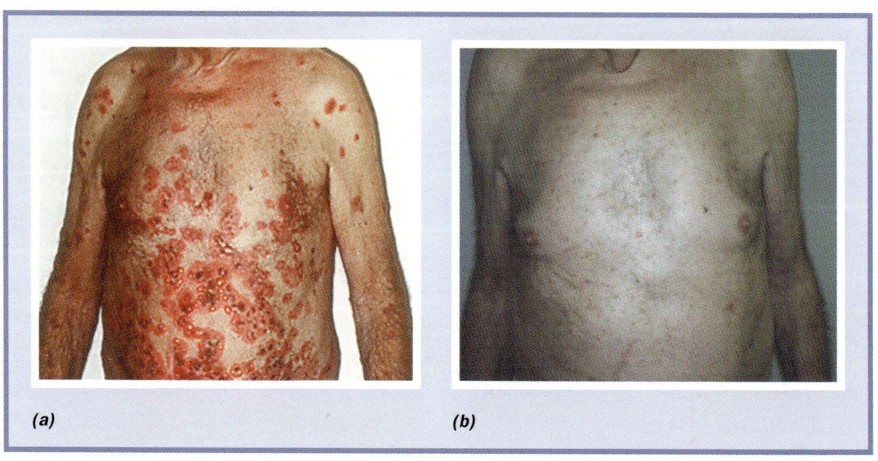



**Fig. 8.5**
*Bullous pemphigoid pre- and post- IVIg therapy. (a) Widespread lesions of bullous pemphigoid pre-IVIg therapy. (b) In the same patient, note complete healing of the lesions post-IVIg therapy.*

used, it is difficult to determine which one is providing clinical recovery. This can also make it difficult to determine the dose and frequency of IVIg therapy. Because BP usually responds to conventional therapy, IVIg has been used in a subgroup of patients who have failed the former. There may therefore be little benefit in continuing adjunctive therapy when it has been ineffective, although this remains to be formally tested.

BP has also been observed to respond faster than other autoimmune blistering diseases and so the number of cycles and duration of treatment required is smaller than for other autoimmune blistering diseases such as PV and PF. IVIg therapy which is gradually tapered has been shown to produce a prolonged sustained clinical remission.[35]

# Cicatricial pemphigoid (mucous membrane pemphigoid)

Cicatricial pemphigoid (CP), also known as mucous membrane pemphigoid, is a severe autoimmune blistering disease with an average age of onset of 62 years.[1] This disease primarily affects the mucous membranes of the oral cavity, conjunctiva, nose, larynx, esophagus, anus and genitalia. Recent studies have demonstrated the presence of autoantibodies to human $\beta_4$-integrin, human $\alpha_6$-integrin, BP Ag 2 and laminin 5.[36–39] In patients who are not treated early in the

course of the disease or who fail to respond to the conventional systemic treatments, CP can progress to potential irreversible damage from scarring. This progression in the eye can result in complete blindness, and in the larynx, sudden asphyxiation due to laryngeal stenosis. In such patients IVIg has become a valuable new addition in the armamentarium of therapy.

There are four large case series and two case reports describing the successful use of IVIg therapy in CP.[40–45] IVIg has been used in the majority of patients after they were observed to be non-responsive to multiple agents used in conventional therapies. The dose and initial frequency of IVIg therapy varied with the severity and aggressive nature of the disease. Patients who have severe cicatricial pemphigoid with predominant involvement of the conjunctiva, are referred to as having ocular cicatricial pemphigoid.[40] In 1999, we reported a group of 10 patients who were blind in one eye as a consequence of progressive CP, and had developed partial involvement of the other eye despite aggressive therapy with multiple immunosuppressive agents. In these patients, IVIg doses of 2–3 g/kg per cycle, given every 2 weeks, were effective in arresting the progression of the disease.[40] The need for a higher dose was confirmed when disease relapse was observed during an acute shortage of IVIg in the United States, and the patients received one-third of their previous dose. However, when

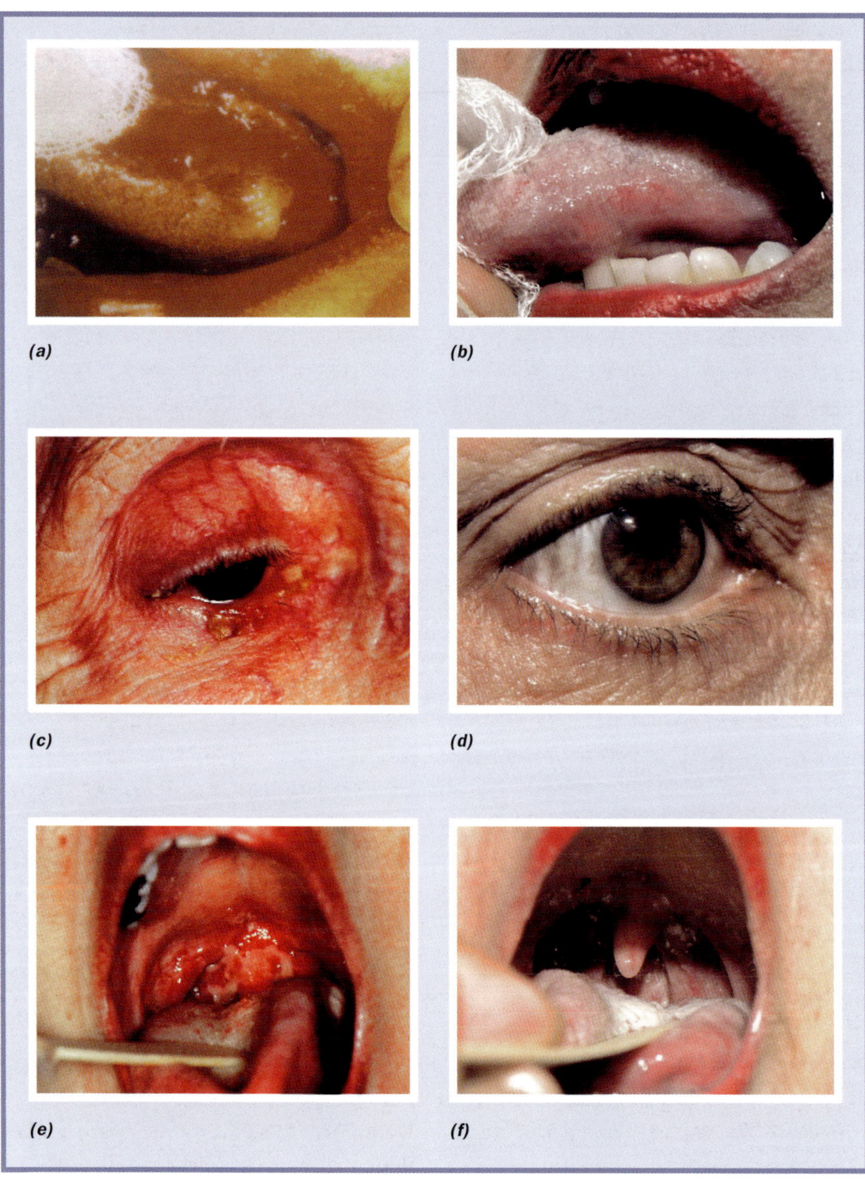

(a)

(b)

(c)

(d)

(e)

(f)

the supply of IVIg resumed and the previous dose was reinstituted, effective clinical control was re-established (Fig. 8.6).

Oral involvement in CP can also be very severe and is referred to as oral pemphigoid (OP).[42,45] Chronic recurrent disease in the oral cavity can also lead to fibrosis of oral tissues, making activities such as eating very difficult. Another major concern in OP is that about 50% of patients develop extraoral involvement when treatment is delayed. Hence, early intervention is necessary. In patients with OP the dose used is 1–2 g/kg per cycle, given initially every 4 weeks.[42,45] In a comparatative study long-term IVIg therapy has been shown to provide effective clinical control in patients with severe OP and to limit disease to the oral cavity (Fig. 8.6).[42] In contrast, patients who were treated with systemic corticosteroids and immunosuppressive agents had frequent relapses, extraoral involvement, severe side-effects, and less than optimal control of clinical disease.[42]

Once an effective response is established, the interval between IVIg infusions is gradually prolonged.[42,45] Abrupt cessation of therapy usually results in relapse of the disease. The frequency of infusions between each cycle is gradually increased to every 6, 8, 10, 12, 14 and 16 weeks. If patients are receiving other systemic conventional treatments, these medications are slowly withdrawn. If patients are disease free at a 16-week interval between two cycles, and off all systemic agents, this is considered the endpoint of therapy. In long-term follow-up, IVIg therapy has been able to induce and maintain long-term clinical remission.

## Epidermolysis bullosa acquisita

Epidermolysis bullosa acquisita (EBA) is an acquired, chronic subepidermal blistering disease characterized by lesions involving the skin and mucous membranes of the eyes, nose, oral cavity, larynx, esophagus and urogenitial tract. EBA lesions on the skin present in the areas of the body which are easily traumatized, such as elbows, knees, and the extensor surfaces of the hands. The sera of patients with EBA have autoantibodies to type

---

**Fig. 8.6**
*Mucous membrane pemphigoid pre- and post-IVIg therapy on the same sites in three different patients. (a) Large erosive lesions on the left lateral border of the tongue and at the junction of the tongue and sublingual mucosa pre-IVIg therapy. (b) In the same patient, resolution of the tongue lesions post-IVIg therapy. (c) Right eye prior to receiving IVIg therapy. Note intense erythema, increased lacrimation, and erosive lesion on the lower eyelid margin, from the midline to the inner canthus. (d) The right eye of the same patient post-IVIg therapy. Note the absence of conjunctival inflammation and the lack of scarring. (e) Erosive lesions involving the entire soft palate pre-IVIg therapy. (f) In the same patient, note the complete healing and resolution of the lesions on the soft palate post-IVIg therapy.*

VII collagen.[46] EBA is a difficult and challenging disease to treat. Although there are different conventional systemic treatments available they are usually only effective with the inflammatory form of EBA and have a number of side-effects. In patients with the mechanobullous non-inflammatory form, these agents do not provide long-term clinical relief. IVIg has recently been shown to be effective in patients who are refractory to other conventional systemic agents.[21,47–54]

IVIg therapy has been shown to be promising in the treatment of EBA. There are eight reports in the literature that have described the successful use of IVIg in eight patients.[21,47–54] These patients had severe disease which was of long duration and recalcitrant to high doses of systemic corticosteroids and multiple immunosuppressive agents.

Patients with severe disease may not respond to cytotoxic agents such as high-dose cyclosporin and cyclophosphamide. In such patients the mean dose of IVIg that has been shown to be effective is 2 g/kg per cycle. In only one patient has low-dose IVIg therapy been clinically effective when all other agents have been discontinued. These cycles have been administered at a frequency of every 4 weeks, and all other systemic agents have been discontinued. Hence, IVIg therapy may then be used as monotherapy. The intervals between cycles can be prolonged as pre-existing lesions heal and no new blister formation is observed, as described in other blistering diseases.

The duration of remissions induced by IVIg in EBA patients is not clearly known because of a lack of long-term follow-up. There are three patients under the care of the authors who have remained free of clinical disease for periods ranging between 4 months and 2 years. Therefore, it is the recommendation of the authors that IVIg therapy be gradually tapered until an endpoint is achieved. Patients need definitive instructions and advice on supportive therapy and strategies to reduce skin trauma. They may require significant lifestyle modifications to achieve such goals.

## Linear IgA bullous disease

Linear IgA bullous disease (LABD) is an autoimmune subepidermal bullous disease characterized by linear IgA deposition along the basement membrane zone.[55–58] The incidence has been reported to be 1 in 200,000.[55] The mean age of onset is 60 years. The lesions generally have a central distribution and can often clinically resemble bullous pemphigoid. LABD has been associated with various malignancies, infections and drugs. Recent studies have identified target antigens in LABD with varying molecular weights, including 97, 120, 180 and 285 kDa proteins.[56–58] Dapsone and sulfapyridine are effective first-line agents in the treatment of LABD. Patients who are recalcitrant to these drugs often require alternative agents.[59–61]

There are three cases in the literature that have described the use of IVIg therapy in LABD. These patients were unresponsive to a combination of different conventional systemic therapies, including systemic corticosteroids, anti-inflammatory and immunosuppressive agents. The dose of IVIg where effective clinical relief was seen ranged between 1 and 2 g/kg per cycle, given initially every 3–4 weeks over 3–5 consecutive days. Patients generally have disease recurrence after 2–3 weeks of IVIg therapy. However, the duration of effective response has varied between 10–12 days and 4–8 weeks. Initially therapy may need to be given at a minimum frequency of every 3 weeks. If patients have recurrences during the second week after IVIg therapy, one infusion can be administered each week while maintaining the total monthly dose. Once no new lesions are observed the frequency between the single weekly infusions can be gradually tapered, with infusions every 2, 3, 4, 6, 8, 10, 12, 14 and 16 weeks. This protocol may allow patients to achieve a sustained clinical remission.

## Herpes gestationis

Herpes gestationis (HG) is an autoimmune disease that usually presents in the second or third trimester of pregnancy or during the immediate postpartum period.[1,55] The disease is characterized by various presentations, from localized involvement of the abdomen and thighs to generalized involvement of the face, palms, soles, chest and back. The disease can be exacerbated at the time of delivery. There is an associated risk of premature delivery and small-for-gestational-age infants. In some cases, neonatal herpes gestationis is the result of transplacental passive transfer of the herpes gestationis autoantibody. The bullae are subepidermal in location and the histology and immunopathology are identical to those of bullous pemphigoid.[55,62] The herpes gestationis autoantigen is also called the HG factor.[62] In recent studies this autoantigen has been demonstrated to be identical to BP Ag2 or one of its epitopes.[62]

The disease usually resolves soon after delivery of the baby. During pregnancy, the disease is treated with topical corticosteroids and systemic antihistamines. In some patients with severe disease, systemic corticosteroids are necessary. If the disease continues to be recalcitrant, treatment options are extremely limited. Although plasmapharesis, cyclophosphamide and cyclosporin all have been reported to be beneficial, they have a high risk of potential irreversible side-effects which could harm both the mother and the fetus.

There is only one case report in the world literature describing the use of IVIg therapy in herpes gestationis.[63] In this case multiple cycles of IVIg therapy were needed to control the disease. IVIg would be an ideal therapy during pregnancy and in the postpartum period, as it is very safe and there are no long-term reported side-effects. It can be used as monotherapy if given frequently, especially near the time of delivery and in the immediate postpartum period. Furthermore, it could possibly prevent the fetus from developing neonatal herpes gestationis. IVIg therapy appears to be a useful option in the management of severe herpes gestationis.

## Side-effects of IVIg therapy

The incidence of side-effects of IVIg therapy is low and they are generally reversible and easily managed. Many side-effects are related to dose, rate of infusion, and the technologies used in the manufacturing process.[64] During the infusions vital signs must be carefully monitored. This is especially crucial as many patients are elderly and usually have several medical problems. Hypertension and congestive heart failure can result from the large fluid volume, especially in patients with compromised cardiac function and borderline renal abnormalities.

The most common side-effects are flushing, myalgia, headache, fever, chills, low backache, nausea or vomiting, chest tightness, wheezing, changes in blood pressure and tachycardia. The most serious include impairment of renal function (especially on a background of existing renal impairment, diabetes and old age), aseptic meningitis and anaphylaxis, especially in patients who have anti-IgA antibodies and are IgA deficient. These side-effects can be avoided by careful screening of patients prior to administering IVIg therapy. There is a very small potential risk of infection with the newer IVIg products, and patients need to be informed of this possibility as well as other possible side-effects. It is worth noting that HIV has never been reported to be transmitted by IVIg.

Before the administration of IVIg therapy patients should undergo thorough blood screening to avoid certain side-effects. Tests should include a complete blood count, renal function tests and immunoglobulin levels, especially IgA. Recently, there have been a number of reports of thromboembolic complications, the cause of which is unclear. However, screening for factors that would enhance hypercoagulability may be advised.

It is interesting that there have been no major side-effects in patients receiving IVIg therapy in blistering diseases. Most side-effects that have been reported have resolved with minimal or no medical intervention.

## Mechanisms of action and autoantibody titers

There are a number of possible mechanisms of action, which have been described in the literature[65] and Chapter 1 but the exact mechanism of action of IVIg in autoimmune blistering diseases is unclear.

One of the major mechanisms is an anti-inflammatory effect through the inhibition of cytokine production.[66,67] One of the cytokines that appears to play an important role in the pathogenesis of pemphigus and pemphigoid is interleukin-1 (IL-1). IL-1$\alpha$ and IL $-1\beta$ are two biochemically distinct forms which have an equal affinity for IL-1 receptors. The inflammatory response that results from these cytokines is competitively inhibited by IL-1 receptor antagonists (IL-1Ra). In patients with PV and CP IVIg upregulates the production of IL-Ra and decreases the production of both IL-1 $\alpha$ and IL-1$\beta$, thereby providing anti-inflammatory effect.[66,67]

There are also different target antigens that have been identified in the various autoimmune blistering diseases. Autoantibody titers to the different target antigens can be measured using serological assays such as indirect immunofluorescence, immunoblotting, and ELISA.[11,68,69] In pemphigus vulgaris, pemphigus foliaceus, bullous pemphigoid, cicatricial pemphigoid and LABD, autoantibody titers have been shown to correlate with disease activity, severity and response to treatment.[45,59,69–72]

In patients treated with IVIg a decline in autoantibody titers has been observed in pemphigus, BP, CP and LABD.[45,59,70–72] The decline has been observed over a long-term follow-up with the specific autoantibody titers. The fall in these titers has correlated with the clinical response to therapy. These observations would suggest that the mechanism(s) of action of IVIg in the blistering diseases may involve effects on the production of pathogenic autoantibodies, as well as effects on the idiotypic–anti-idiotypic network. The combination of mechanisms involved could result in the restoration of the immune network and hence a clinical remission. Further experimental studies are needed to define these exact mechanism(s) of action of IVIg in autoimmune blistering diseases.

## Conclusion

From the initial studies it is evident that IVIg therapy is an effective alternative in the treatment of autoimmune blistering diseases. There are general conclusions which can be drawn from these outcome studies.

IVIg therapy may not be the treatment of choice in every patient with autoimmune blistering diseases. The potential indications for IVIg therapy in autoimmune blistering diseases fall into a a number of categories: (1) patients who are unresponsive to conventional local and systemic treatments; (2) patients in whom conventional systemic therapy has produced debilitating side-effects; (3) contraindications to the use of conventional systemic treatments; and (4) patients with severe disease.

The major limitation in these studies is they are not case-control trials and do not consist of large numbers of patients. However, in view of the rarity of these conditions it is difficult to design large, appropriately powered studies in the absence of multicenter involvement. Therefore, until such trials are available, the recommended protocols are those that have been published. Because of the extent and severity of these diseases, high-dose IVIg therapy in a total dose ranging between 1 and 2 g/kg per treatment cycle is necessary at a minimum initial frequency interval of 3–4 weeks between cycles. It is also evident that multiple cycles are generally required to achieve disease control. A great advantage of long-term IVIg therapy is that it may permit the discontinuation of systemic agents, and hence can be eventually used as monotherapy.

The conventional agents have not only failed to provide a good clinical response, but have also provided a poor quality of life because of their short- and long-term side-effects. IVIg therapy provides a significant improvement in the quality of life as there are minimal side-effects and effective control of disease progression is established.

Because IVIg is a promising new therapy, with minimal side-effects and significant clinical benefits, it is essential to organize and conduct multicenter trials. Such trials will help in developing accurate defined and

agreed-upon clinical outcome parameters, changes in protocol if necessary, and expand the spectrum of indications for usage. IVIg heralds a new era for the treatment of blistering diseases with biological products that focus on immune reconstitution and not on conventional immune suppression. In the future, we can expect that as the process of immune dysfunction is better understood, we may be able to identify and focus upon exactly which molecule(s) hold the key to pathogenesis and hence recovery. IVIg opens the door for these and other possible investigations and research.

## References


1. Scott JE, Ahmed AR, The blistering diseases. *Med Clin North Am* 1998; **82**: 1239–83.

2. Savin JA. The events leading to the death of patients with pemphigus and pemphigoid. *Br J Dermatol* 1979; **101**: 521–34.

3. Lever WF. Pemphigus and pemphigoid. *J Am Acad Dermatol* 1979; **1**: 2–31.

4. Ahmed AR, Moy R. Death in pemphigus. *J Am Acad Dermtol* 1982; **7**: 221–8.

5. Bystryn JC, Steinman NM. The adjuvant therapy of pemphigus. *Arch Dermatol* 1996; **132**: 203–12.

6. Holloran PF. Immunosuppressive agents in clinical trials in transplantation. *Am J Med Sci* 1997; **313**: 283–8.

7. Grundmann-Kollmann M, Korting HC, Behrens S et al. Mycophenolate mofetil: a new therapeutic option in the treatment of

blistering autoimmune diseases. *J Am Acad Dermatol* 1999; **40**: 957–60.

8.  Briggs JD. A criticial review of immunosuppressive therapy. *Immunol Lett* 1991; **29**: 89–94.

9.  Otley CC. Immunosuppression and skin cancer: pathogenetic insights, therapeutic challenges, and opportunities for innovation. *Arch Dermatol* 2002; **138**: 827–8.

10. Jolles S, Hughes J, Whittaker S. Dermatological uses of high-dose intravenous immunoglobulin. *Arch Dermatol* 1998; **134**: 80–6.

11. Beutner EH, Jordan RE, Chorzelski TP. The immunopathology of pemphigus and bullous pemphigoid. *J Invest Dermatol* 1968; **51**: 63–8.

12. Amagai M, Tsunoda K, Zillikens D, Nagai T, Nishikawa T. The clinical phenotype of pemphigus is defined by the anti-desmoglein autoantibody profile. *J Am Acad Dermatol* 1999; **40**: 167–70.

13. Carson PJ, Hameed A, Ahmed AR. Influence of treatment on the clinical course of pemphigus vulgaris. *J Am Acad Dermatol* 1996; **34**: 645–52.

14. Tappeniner G, Steiner A. High-dosage intravenous immunoglobulin: therapeutic failure in pemphigus and pemphigoid. *J Am Acad Dermatol* 1989; **20**: 684–5.

15. Humbert P, Derancourt C, Aubin F, Agache P. Effects of intravenous gamma globulin in pemphigus. *J Am Acad Dermatol* 1990; **22**: 326.

16. Messer G, Sizmann N, Feucht H, Meurer M. High-dose intravenous immunoglobulins for immediate control of severe pemphigus vulgaris. *Br J Dermatol* 1995; **133**: 1014–15.

17. Beckers RCY, Brand A, Vermeer BJ, Boom BW. Adjuvant high-dose intravenous immunoglobulins in the treatment of pemphigus and bullous pemphigoid: experience in six patients. *Br J Dermatol* 1995; **133**: 289–93.

18. Bewely AP, Keefe M. Successful treatment of pemphigus vulgaris by pulsed intravenous immunoglobulin therapy. *Br J Dermatol* 1996; **135**: 128–9.

19. Wever S, Zillikens D, Brocker EB. Successful treatment of refractory mucosal lesions of pemphigus vulgaris using intravenous gammaglobulin as adjuvant therapy. *Br J Dermatol* 1996; **135**: 852–6.

20. Colonna L, Cianchini F, Frezzolini A, De Pita O, Lella G, Puddu P. Intravenous immunoglobulins for pemphigus vulgaris: adjuvant vs first choice therapy. *Br J Dermatol* 1998; **138**: 1102–3.

21. Harman KE, Black MM. High-dose intravenous immunoglobulin for the treatment of autoimmune blistering diseases: an evaluation of its use in 14 cases. *Br J Dermatol* 1999; **140**: 865–74.

22. Jolles S, Huges J, Rustin M. Therapeutic failure of high-dose intravenous immunoglobulin in pemphigus vulgaris. *J Am Acad Dermatol* 1999; **40**: 499–500.

23. Ahmed AR. Intravenous immunoglobulin therapy in the treatment of patients with pemphigus vulgaris unresponsive to conventional immunosuppressive treatment. *J Am Acad Dermatol* 2001; **45**: 679–90.

24. Sami N, Qureshi A, Ruocco E, Ahmed AR. Corticosteroid-sparing effect of intravenous immunoglobulin therapy in patients with pemphigus vulgaris. *Arch Dermatol* 2002; **138**: 58–62.

25. Sami N, Bhol K, Ahmed AR. Diagnostic features of pemphigus vulgaris in patients with pemphigus foliaceus: detection of both autoantibodies, long-term follow-up, and treatment responses. *Clin Exp Immunol* 2001; **125**: 492–8.

26. Azana JM, de Misa RF, Harto A, Ledo A. Severe pemphigus foliaceus treated with extracorporeal photochemotherapy. *Arch Dermatol* 1997; **133**: 287–9.

27. Cintin C, Joffe P. Pemphigus foliaceus treated successfully with plasma exchange. *Int J Dermatol* 1992; **31**: 871–2.

28. Ahmed AR, Sami N. Intravenous immunoglobulin therapy for patients with pemphigus foliaceus unresponsive to conventional therapy. *J Am Acad Dermatol* 2002; **46**: 42–9.

29. Sami N, Qureshi A, Ahmed AR. Steroid sparing effect of intravenous immunoglobulin therapy in patients with pemphigus foliaceus. *Eur J Dermatol* 2002; **12**: 174–8.

30. Toth GG, Jonkman MF. Successful treatment of recalcitrant penicillamine-induced pemphigus foliaceus by low-dose intravenous immunoglobulins. *Br J Dermatol* 1999; **141**: 583–5.

31. Stanely JR, Hawley-Nelson P, Yuspa SH et al. Characterization of bullous pemphigoid antigen: a unique basement membrane protein of stratified squamous epithelia. *Cell* 1981; **24**: 897.

32. Labib RS, Anhalt GJ, Patel HP et al. Molecular heterogeneity of the bullous pemphigoid antigens as detected by immunoblotting. *J Immunol* 1986; **136**: 1231.

33. Godard W, Roujeau JC, Guillot B, Andre C, Rifle G. Bullous pemphigoid and intravenous immunoglobulin. *Ann Intern Med* 1985; **103**: 964–5.

34. Engineer L, Ahmed AR. Role of intravenous immunoglobulin in the treatment of bullous pemphigoid: analysis of current data. *J Am Acad Dermatol* 2001; **44**: 83–8.

35. Ahmed AR. Intravenous immunoglobulin therapy for patients with bullous pemphigoid unresponsive to conventional immunosuppressive treatment. *J Am Acad Dermatol* 2001; **45**: 825–35.

36. Domloge-Hultsch N, Anhalt GJ, Gammon WR et al. Aniepilgirin cicatricial pemphigoid. A subepithelial disorder. *Arch Dermatol* 1994; **130**: 1521–9.

37. Balding SD, Prost C, Diaz L et al. Cicatricial pemphigoid autoantibodies react with multiple sites on the BP extracellular domain. *J Invest Dermatol* 1996; **106**: 141–6.

38. Bhol KC, Goss L, Kumari S, Colon JE, Ahmed AR. Autoantibodies to human alpha 6 integrin patients with oral pemphigoid. *J Dent Res* 2001; **80**: 1711–15.

39. Chan R, Bhol KC, Tesavibul N et al. The role of human B4 integrin in conjunctival basement membrane separation. Possible in vitro model for OCP. *Invest Ophthalmol Vis Sci* 1999; **30**: 2283–90.

40. Foster CS, Ahmed AR. Intravenous immunoglobulin therapy for ocular cicatricial pemphigoid: a preliminary study. *Ophthalmology* 1999; **106**: 2136–43.

41. Urcelay ML, McQueen A, Douglas WS. Cicatricial pemphigoid treated with intravenous immunoglobulin. *Br J Dermatol* 1997; **137**: 477–8.

42. Ahmed AR, Colon JE. Comparison between intravenous immunoglobulin and conventional immunosuppressive therapy

regimens in patients with severe oral pemphigoid. *Arch Dermatol* 2001; **137**: 1181–9.

43.   Sami N, Bhol KC, Ahmed AR. Intravenous immunoglobulin therapy in patients with multiple mucosal involvement in mucous membrane pemphigoid. *Clin Immunol* 2002; **102**: 59–67.

44.   Leverkus M, Georgi M, Nie Z, Hashimoto T, Brocker EB, Zillkens D. Cicatricial pemphigoid with circulation IgA and IgG autoantibodies to the central portion of the BP 180 ectodomain: beneficial effect of adjuvant therapy with high-dose intravenous immunoglobulin. *J Am Acad Dermatol* 2002; **46**: 116–22.

45.   Sami N, Bhol KC, Ahmed AR. Treatment of oral pemphigoid with intravenous immunoglobulin as monotherapy long-term follow-up: influence of treatment on autoantibody titers to human alpha 6 integrin. *Clin Exp Immunol* 2002; **129**: 533–40.

46.   Woodely DT, Briggaman RA, O'Keefe EJ et al. Indentification of the skin basement membrane autoantigen in epidermolysis bullosa acquisita. *N Engl J Med* 1984; **310**: 1007–14.

47.   Meir F, Sonnichsen K, Scaumber-Lever G, Dopfer R, Rassner G. Epidermolysis bullosa acquisita:efficacy of high dose intravenous immunoglobulins. *J Am Acad Dermatol* 1993; **29**: 334–7.

48.   Caldwell JB, Yancey KB, Engler RJM, James WD. Epidermolysis bullosa acquisita: efficacy of high dose intravenous immunoglobulins. *J Am Acad Dermatol* 1994; **31**: 827–8.

49.   Mohr C, Sunderkotter C, Hildebran A et al. Successful treatment of Epidermolysis Bullosa Acquisita using intravenous immunoglobulins. *Br J Dermatol* 1995; **132**: 824–6.

50.   Kofler H, Wambacher-Gasser B, Topar G et al. Intravneous immunoglobulin treatment in therapy-resistant epidermolysis bullosa acquisita. *J Am Acad Dermatol* 1996; **34**: 331–5.

51.   Harman KE, Whittam LR, Wakeling SH, Black MM. Severe refractory epidermolysis bullosa complicated by an oesophageal stricture responding to intravenous immune globulin. *Br J Dermatol* 1998; **139**: 1126–7.

52.   Jappe U, Zillikens D, Bonnekoh B, Gollnick H. Epidermolysis bullosa acquisita with ultraviolet radiation sensitivity. *Br J Dermatol* 2000; **142**: 517–20.

53.   Engineer L, Ahmed AR. Emerging treatment for epidermolysis bullosa acquisita. *J Am Acad Dermatol* 2001; **44**: 818–28.

54.   Engineer L, Ahmed AR. Epidermolysis bullosa acquisita and multiple myeloma. *J Am Acad Dermatol* 2002; (in press).

55.   Jordan RE. *Atlas of Bullous Disease.* Philadelphia: Churchill Livingstone, 2000.

56.   Wojnarowska F, Allen J, Collier P. Linear IgA disease: a heterogeneous disease. *Dermatology* 1994; **18**: 52–6.

57.   Pas HH, Kloosterhuis GJ, Heeres K, van deer Meer JM, Jonkman MF. Bullous pemphigoid and linear IgA dermatosis sera recognize a similar 120 kDa keratinocyte collagenous glycoprotein with antigenic cross reactivity to BP 180; *J Invest Dermatol* 1997; **108**: 423–9.

58.   Chan LS, Tracyk T, Tayler TB, Eramo LR, Woodley DT, Zone JJ. Linear IgA bullous dermatosis. Characterization of a subset of patients with concurrent IgA and IgG antibasement membrane autoantibodies. *Arch Dermatol* 1995; **131**: 1432–7.

59.   Khan IU, Bhol KC Ahmed AR. Linear IgA bullous dermatosis in a patient with chronic renal failure: response to intravenous immunoglobulin therapy. *J Am Acad Dermatol* 1999; **40:** 485–8.

60.   Kroiss M, Vogt T, Landthaler M, Stolz W. High-dose intravenous immunoglobulin is also effective in linear IgA disease. *Br J Dermatol* 2000; **142:** 582.

61.   Letko E, Bhol K, Foster CS, Ahmed AR. Linear IgA bullous disease limited to the eye: a diagnostic dilemma: response to intravenous immunoglobulin therapy. *Ophthalmology.* 2000; **107:** 1524–8.

62.   Kelly SE, Bhogal BS, Wojnarowska F, Black MM. Expression of a pemphigoid gestationis-related antigen by human placenta. *Br J Dermatol* 1988; **118:** 605–11.

63.   Hern S, Harman K, Bhogal BS, Black MM. A severe persistent case of pemphigoid gestationis treated with intravenous immunoglobulins and cyclosporin. *Clin Exp Dermatol* 1998; **23:** 185–8.

64.   Mobini N, Sarela A, Ahmed AR. Intravenous immunoglobulins in the therapy of autoimmune and systemic inflammatory disorders. *Ann Allergy Asthma Immunol* 1995; **74:** 119–32.

65.   Kazatchkine MD, Kaveri SV. Immunomodulation of autoimmune and inflammatory diseases with intravenous immune globulin. *N Engl J Med* 2001; **345:** 747–55.

66.   Bhol KC, Desai A, Kumari S, Colon JE,

Ahmed AR. Pemphigus vulgaris: the role of IL-1 and IL-1 receptor antagonist in pathogenesis and effects of intravenous immunoglobulin on their production. *Clin Immunol* 2001; **100:** 172–80.

67.   Kumari S, Bhol KC, Rehman F, Foster CS, Ahmed AR. Interleukin 1 components in cicatricial pemphigoid. Role in intravenous immunoglobulin therapy. *Cytokine* 2001; **14:** 218–24.

68.   Bhol K, Tyagi S, Natarajan K, Nagarwalla N, Ahmed AR. Use of recombinant pemphigus vulgaris antigen in the development of ELISA and IB assays to detect pemphigus vulgaris autoantibodies. *J Eur Acad Dermatol Venereol* 1998; **10:** 28–35.

69.   Amagai M, Komai A, Hashimoto T et al. Usefulness of enzyme-linked immunosorbent assay using recombinant desmogleins 1 and 3 for serodiagnosis of pemphigus. *Br J Dermatol* 1999; **140:** 351–7.

70.   Schmidt E, Obe K, Brocker EB, Zillikens D. Serum levels of autoantibodies to BP 180 correlate with disease activity in patients with bullous pemphigoid. *Arch Dermatol* 2000; **136:** 174–8.

71.   Letko E, Bhol KC, Foster CS, Ahmed AR. Influence of intravenous immunoglobulin therapy on serum levels of anti-B4 antibodies in ocular cicatricial pemphigoid. *Curr Eye Res* 2000; **21:** 646–54.

72.   Sami N, Bhol KC, Ahmed AR. Influence of IVIg therapy on autoantibody titers to desmoglein 1 in patients with pemphigus foliaceus. *Clin Immunol* 2002; (in press).

# Safety and tolerability of intravenous immunoglobulins

**Turf D Martin**

IVIg, intravenous immunoglobulin; TTV, transfusion transmitted virus; vCJD, variant Creutzfeld–Jacob disease; PCR, polymerase chain reaction

## Introduction

Intravenous immunoglobulin (IVIg) is derived from human plasma by recovery from whole blood donors or by plasmapheresis. Prior to 1981, only products that had a modified Fc function were commercially available from manufacturers. These products were used in a limited manner for immune replacement in patients with defective IgG. The second-generation products, with an intact Fc function, have allowed the use of IVIg for broader immune replacement therapy in patients with defective B-cell function(s) and in immune modulation. This has resulted in the significant increase in the use of IVIg in autoimmune disorders, including those in dermatology. Current applications include dermatomyositis, Kawasaki's disease, bullous pemphigoid, linear IgA, ocular cicatricial pemphigoid, toxic epidermal necrolysis, chronic urticaria and atopic dermatitis.

**Table 9.1**
IVIg Information chart

| PRODUCT | Aventis Behring | Novartis/AmRed Cross ZLB/CSL | Aventis Behring | Immuno Baxter | Aventis Behring | Baxter/Hyland Am.Red Cross | PRODUCT |
|---|---|---|---|---|---|---|---|
| Name(s) | Gamma-Venin P | Sandoglobulin Panglobulin Careimune | Venimmun | Endobulin | Gammar PIV Armoglobulina | Gammagard SD Polyglobulin | Name(s) |
| Manufactured in | Germany | Switzerland | Germany | Austria | USA | USA/Belgium | Country of manf |
| Process | Cohn | Kistler-Nitschmann pH4, pepsin nanofiltration | Cohn Sulfitolysis | Cohn PEG | Cohn pH4 | Cohn DEAE Sephadex PEG | Process |
| Plasma source | German | US/Swiss | German | US/Aus/Ger | US | US | Plasma source |
| Type | 5s | 7s | 7s | 7s | 7s | 7s | Type |
| Form | powder | powder | powder | powder | powder | powder | Form |
| Viral inactivation | Pastereurized | pH4 | Past. | SD | Past. | SD | Viral inactivatio |
| Concentration | 5% | 3–12% | 5% | 5% | 5–10% | 5–10% | Concentration |
| Half-life (days) | 12–36 hours | 30 | 21–36 | 27 | 22 | 24 | Half-life (days) |
| % IgG | >95 | >96 | >85 | >99 | >98 | >99 | % IgG |
| $IgG_1$ % | | 65.2 | 65 | 60–70 | 69 | 71.2 | $IgG_1$ % |
| $IgG_2$ % | | 28.3 | 25 | 30-40 | 23 | 21.3 | $IgG_2$ % |
| $IgG_3$ % | | 4.15 | 5 | 0.8 | 6 | 4.5 | $IgG_3$ % |
| $IgG_4$ % | | 2.4 | 5 | 2 | 2 | 3.1 | $IgG_4$ % |
| % Monomers | >95 | 86 | >80 | <93 | >90 | >90 | % Monomers |
| % Dimers | | >4% | >10% | | | | % Dimers |
| IgA (mg/ml) | | 1.2 | 5 | 0.06 | <0.1 | <0.003 | IgA (mg/ml) |
| IgM (mg/ml) | | <0.1 | | <0.1 | <0.1 | <0.1 | IgM (mg/ml) |
| Sodium (mg/ml) | 8.5 | 9 | 8.5 | 3 | 5 | 9 | Sodium (mg/ml) |
| Sugar/stabilizer | Glycine | Sucrose | Glycine | Glucose | Sucrose | Glucose/glycine | Sugar/stabilizer |
| Osmolality | | 680–1074(NaCl) | | 357 | | | Osmolality |
| Albumin content | none | 3% | none | ? | 8.0 mg/ml | 3 | Albumin content |
| pH | 6.8 | 6.6 | 6.8 | 7 | 7 | 7 | pH |
| Anti-A | | | | | | 1;4 | Anti-A |
| Anti-B | | | | | | 1;8 | Anti-B |
| Anti-D | | | | | | | Anti-D |
| Pkg. sizes | 0.25/0.5/2.5/5/10 | 1/3/6/12 | 0.5/2.5/5/10 | 0.25/0.5/1 2.5/5/7.5/10 | 0.5/2.5/5/10 | 0.5/2.5/5/10 | Pkg sizes |
| Shelf-life (m) | 24 | 36 | 24 | 24 | 24 | 24 | Shelf-life (m) |
| Storage | Room temp | Room temp | Room temp | Refrigerate | Room temp | Room temp | Storage |
| Solubility | | 20 minutes | | | | 3–10 min | |
| Max infusion rate | 2–3 ml/min | 2.5 ml/min | 2 ml/min | 0.33 ml/kg/min | 2.5 ml/min | 0.13 ml/kg/min | Max infusion ra |
| Registration notes | only Germany | worldwide | Germ / Aust | Aust/Germ Switz/USA Italy | USA | worldwide | Registration no |
| Info source Promotional Material | German | French | German | Intl Eng | US | Intl English | Inform source |

| PRODUCT | Bayer/Miles Tropon | Bayer | Octapharma | Bioventrum | BPL | Biotest | Biotest |
|---|---|---|---|---|---|---|---|
| **Name(s)** | Polyglobin 5% Gamimune5% | Polyglobin 10% Gamimune 10% | OCTAGAM | GammoNativ N | Viagam-S | Intraglobin F | Intraglobin CP (chrom.purified) |
| **Country of manuf** | USA | USA | Austria | Sweden | UK | Germany | Germany |
| **Process** | Cohn | Cohn–Oncley | Cohn | Cohn | Cohn | Cohn | Chromatography |
|  | pH4 | pH4 incubation S/D | pH4 | DEAE Sephadex | Ion Exchange | B-propiolactone |  |
| **Plasma source** | US | USA | Aus/Ger/US | Swedish | USA | US/Aus/Ger | US/Aus/Ger/Belg |
| **Type** | 7s | 7s | 7s | 7s | 7s | 7s | 7s |
| **Form** | liquid | liquid | liquid | powder | powder | liquid | liquid |
| **Viral inactivation** | SD/pH4 | SD, pH4, LpH | SD, pH4 | SD | S/D | B-prop./Nanofiltr. | SD/Filtration |
| **Concentration** | 5% | 10% | 5% | 5% | 5% | 5% | 5% |
| **Half-life (days)** | 26.4 | > 21 days | 28 | 20–25 |  | 21.6 | 22 |
| **% IgG** | 98% | > 98% | > 99 |  | > 98 | >95 | > 95 |
| **IgG$_1$ %** | 64.6 | 63.2 | 63 | 60.9 | 51.7 | 59.6 | 59 |
| **IgG$_2$ %** | 28.6 | 29.6 | 28.5 | 35.2 | 40.9 | 36.6 | 36 |
| **IgG$_3$ %** | 5.7 | 5.7 | 6.3 | 3 | 6.4 | 0.4 | 3 |
| **IgG$_4$ %** | 1.1 | 1.3 | 2.7 | 0.9 | 1 | 3.4 | 2 |
| **% Monomers** | > 99 | 99 | > 92 | 96 | 93.3 |  |  |
| **% Dimers** |  | 0 | > 7% |  |  |  |  |
| **IgA (mg/ml)** | <0.21 | <0,2 | <0.1 | <0.002 | 5 | 1.5 | <2.5 |
| **IgM (mg/ml)** | <0.1 |  | <0.1 | <0.1 | <0.1 | <0.1 | <0.1 |
| **Sodium (mg/ml)** | 1.2 |  | 0.01 | 9 | 5.9 |  |  |
| **Sugar/stabilizer** | Maltose | Glycine | Maltose | Glycine/Glucose | Sucrose | Glucose | Glycine |
| **Osmolality** | 336 | 261 | > 250 < 350 | 415 | 340 |  | 300 |
| **Albumin content** | none | none | none | 50 | 20 | none | none |
| **pH** | 4.2 | 4.25 | 5.5–6.0 | 7 | 6.6 |  | 513 |
| **Anti-A** | 1;8 | 1:08 | 1;1 | 1;8 |  |  |  |
| **Anti-B** | 1:02 | 1:04 | 1;1 | 1;16 |  |  |  |
| **Anti-D** |  |  | ND |  |  |  |  |
| **Pkg sizes** | 0.5/2.5/5/10 | 1, 5, 10, 20 | 1.0/2.5/5.0/ 10.0 | 2,5/5 | 2,5/5 | 0.5/1.0/2.5/ 5,0/10 | 1/2.5/5/10 |
| **Shelf-life (m)** | 24 | 36 | 24 | 36 | 24 | 24 | 36 |
| **Storage** | Refrigerate | Refrig. | Room temp. | Refrigerate 8 min | Room temp | Refrigerate | Refrigerate |
| **Max infusion rate** | 0.08 ml/kg/min | 0.08 ml/kg/min | 3 ml/min | 3 ml/min | 3 ml/min | 2 ml/min |  |
| **Registration notes** | worldwide | US/Europe | worldwide | Scand./Germ | UK | Germ/Aus/Switz | Germany |
| **Inform source** | German Intl | US Pkg. Leaf. German Broch. | Intl English | Swedish Intl | UK | German | German |
|  |  |  |  |  |  |  | PEI approved Aug-01 |

**Table 9.1**
continued

| BPL | Griffols | Alpha | Alpha | Biagini | PRODUCT | Kedrion Biagini | LFB |
|---|---|---|---|---|---|---|---|
| Viagam Liquid | Alphaglobin Flebogamma | Venoglobulin S 5% | Venoglobulin S 10% | Biavin | **Name(s)** | Isivin | Tegeline |
| UK | Spain | USA | US | Italy | **Country of manuf** | Italy | France |
| Cohn<br>Ion exchange<br>ph4 Incub | Cohn<br>PEG | Cohn<br>PEG | Cohn<br>PEG | Cohn<br>Ion Exchange | **Process** | Cohn<br>pH4 | Cohn<br>pH4/pepsin |
| USA | US/EC | US | US | Italian | **Plasma source** | Italian | French |
| 7s | 7s | 7s | 7s | 7s | **Type** | 7s | 7s |
| liquid | liquid | liquid | liquid | powder | **Form** | powder | powder |
| SD, pH4 | Pasteruized | SD/pH4 | SD/pH4 | SD | **Viral inactivation** | SD, pH4 | pH4 |
| 5% | 5% | 5% | 10% | 5% | **Concentration** | 5% | 3–12% |
| 21 | 36–65 | 33.5+/–7 | | 24 | **Half-life (days)** | 24 | 24 |
| 100 | >99 | >99 | | | **% IgG** | 99 | >97 |
| 56 | 69.7 | 69.7 | | | **IgG$_1$ %** | 62–70 | 58.8 |
| 38 | 28.13 | 28.2 | | | **IgG$_2$ %** | 20–24 | 34.1 |
| 5.4 | 1.32 | 1.3 | | | **IgG$_3$ %** | 8.6–9.4 | 5.4 |
| 0.6 | 0.87 | 0.9 | | | **IgG$_4$ %** | 3.8–4.2 | 1.7 |
| 95 | | >94 | | | **% Monomers** | 0 | |
| 3.5 | | | | | **% Dimers** | 100 | |
| 5 | <0.05 | <0.008 | | 0.1 | **IgA (mg/ml)** | 0.118 | 0.85 |
| | <0.1 | <0.1 | | <0.1 | **IgM (mg/ml)** | 0.1 | <0.1 |
| 119 mmol/l | | | | 9 | **Sodium (mg/ml)** | 8.5 | 2 |
| sucrose | D-Sorbital | D-Sorbital | D-Sorbital | Sucrose | **Sugar/stabilizer** | Sucrose | Sucrose |
| 400 | | 300 | 330 | | **Osmolality** | 450–600 | |
| 2 g/5g vial | | 1.3 | 2.6 | none | **Albumin content** | none | |
| 4.9 | 5,4 | 5.2–5.8 | | 6.8 | **pH** | 7 | |
| | | 1;8 | | low | **Anti-A** | 1:04 | |
| | | 1;8 | | low | **Anti-B** | 1:04 | |
| | | | | low | **Anti-D** | | |
| 5 | 0,5/2,5/5/10 | 2.5/5/10 | 5/10/20,0 | 0,5/1/2,5/5 | **Pkg Sizes** | 1/2,5/5 | 0,5/2,5/5/10 |
| 24 | 24 | 24 | 24 | 36 | **Shelf-life (m)** | 36 | 36 |
| Refrig | Room temp<br>Refrig in Spain | Room temp | Refrigerate | Room temp | **Storage** | Room temp | Room temp |
| 3 ml/min | | 0.08 ml/kg/min | 0.05 ml/kg/min | | **Max infusion rate** | | 0.067 ml/kg/mi |
| UK | Spain, Port, UK<br>Germ, Switz | USA | USA | Italy | **Registration notes** | Italy | France |
| UK | Spain/Germ | US | US | Turkish | **Inform Source** | Turkish | French |
| | Expanding registrations in export countries, USA, Portugal | sorbital cannot be used for fructose intolerance | | | | | |

All information is derived from manufacturer's sales brochure and package inserts. SD = solvent detergent; Past. = pasturization.

| CLB | BRC | Finnish Red Cross | Human | CSL | PRODUCT | Shanghai Raas | CBSF/BioTrust (Yung Shin Pharm) | Normal Plasma |
|---|---|---|---|---|---|---|---|---|
| See Biotest Intraglobin F | See Biotest Intraglobin F | | Humaglobin | Intragam p | **Name(s)** | Gammaraas | see Sandoglobulin self Sufficiency | |
| Neth | Belg | Finland | Hungary | Australia | **Country of manuf** | China | Taiwan | |
| | | Cohn | Cohn | Cohn/Column | **Process** | Cohn | | |
| | | pH4/pepsin | PEG | | | | | |
| Dutch | Belg | Finnish | Hungary | Australia | **Plasma source** | China | Taiwan | |
| | | 7s | 7s | 7s | **Type** | 7s | 7s | |
| | | liquid | Powder | liquid | **Form** | liquid | powder | |
| | | SD/Nanofilr | Heat | unkown | **Viral inactivation** | double | | |
| 5% | 5% | 5% | 5% | 6% | **Concentration** | 5% | 3% | |
| | | | 22 | | **Half-life (days)** | | | |
| | | | >95 | 21–42 | **% IgG** | | | |
| | | | 68 | | **IgG$_1$ %** | | | 60–70 |
| | | | 29 | | **IgG$_2$ %** | | | 15–25 |
| | | | 1 | | **IgG$_3$ %** | | | 4,0–8 |
| | | | 2 | | **IgG$_4$ %** | | | 2,0–8 |
| | | | | >90 | **% Monomers** | | | |
| | | | | | **% Dimers** | | | |
| | | | <0.05 | | **IgA (mg/ml)** | <0.12 | | |
| | | | | | **IgM (mg/ml)** | | | |
| | | | | | **Sodium (mg/ml)** | | | |
| | | | glucose/glycin | Maltose | **Sugar/stabilizer** | | | |
| | | | >240 | | **Osmolality** | | | 290 |
| | | | | none | **Albumin content** | | | |
| | | | 7.0 | 4.25 | **pH** | | | |
| | | | 1;64 | | **Anti-A** | | | |
| | | | 1;64 | | **Anti-B** | | | |
| | | | | | **Anti-D** | | | |
| | | | 0.5,1,2.5,5 | 6 | **Pkg sizes** | | | |
| | | 24 | | 24 | **Shelf-life (m)** | | | |
| | | Room temp | Refrigerate | Refrigerate | **Storage** | | | |
| | | | 0.01 ml/kg | 4 ml/min | **Max infusion rate** | | | |
| Neth | Belgium | Finland | Hungary | PanPacific | **Registration notes** | | | |
| | | Finland | Hungary | Malysia PI | **Inform source** | | | |

## Pharmacology

IVIg products are not generics nor are considered equivalent. The USA Food and Drug Administration (FDA) considers each biological a new molecule, thereby not allowing their registration as generics. Manufacturers only purify the IgG protein (Fig. 9.1). They cannot improve on what the human body makes, only damage the molecule during purification or through the addition of various excipients. Most adverse reactions are the result of the purification process and/or the addition of excipients. These differences are very evident when the properties are compared side by side. Table 9.1 lists those products available in Europe and the United States. The data are taken directly from the manufacturers' own promotional literature and package leaflets.

The critical question is whether a clinical failure is due to the failure of IgG or the failure of a specific product that is not of the highest purification quality. Because of the cost, many pharmacies and buying groups purchase IVIg as generics, taking only the price into consideration. The products are patented only by the purification process, not the 'drug'. Technology has advanced considerably in the last 20 years, resulting in much higher purity and molecular integrity than previously, yet the older products remain on the market and are often sold as commodity products, differentiated only by

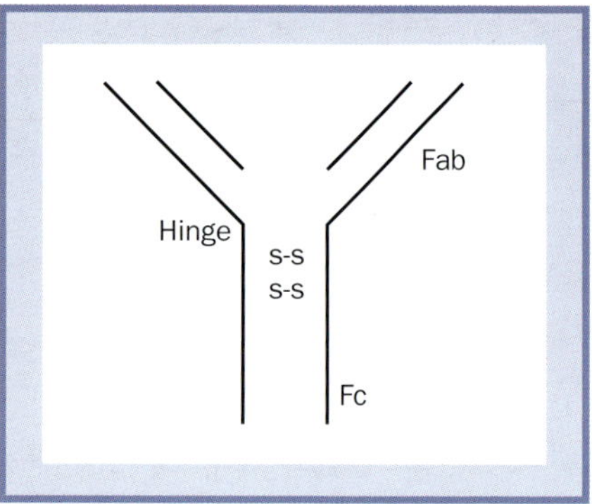


**Fig. 9.1**
*The IgG molecule*

lower prices. Modern technology does cost more.

IgG is produced by the humoral portion of the human immune system, i.e. B cells. As such, it has an extensive function as an immune modulator. Various mechanisms of action have been proposed for its many clinical applications. These include Fc-receptor mediator effects, suppression of superantigens, upregulation of anti-inflammatory cytokines and downregulation of inflammatory cytokines, neutralization of alloantibodies (anti-idiotypic effect), and the selection of immune repertoires. Many other mechanisms continue to be researched.

## Virological safety

Because IVIg is a plasma derivative, concern has been expressed about the potential for virus transmission. Viruses that are of concern are the transfusion-related viruses such as hepatitis A, B and C, HIV, HTLV I/II, cytomegalovirus, human herpes virus, and parvovirus $B_{19}$. Another pathogen of concern is the variant Creutzfeld–Jakob disease prion (vCJD).

Reports of non-A, non-B hepatitis transmission have been published since 1983.[1–6] In 1994, transmission of hepatitis C was reported in 247 patients receiving Gammagard*.[7]

Other agents have recently become of concern, including Creuzfeldt–Jakob, transfusion transmitted virus (TTV) and hepatitis G. Viral safety with IVIg begins with the donor and the donor center, i.e. the starting material. In Europe and North America, all centers must meet either European Community (EC) and/or Food and Drug Administration (FDA) criteria. In North America, some donor centers qualify for a program administered by the American Blood Resources Organization (ABRA) called the Quality Plasma Program (QPP), which sets higher standards than even those of the FDA. European manufacturers obtain their plasma from the United States and/or Europe (usually Austria and Germany, unless the company is nationally controlled or has

*Gammagard is a registered trademark of Baxter Healthcare Corporation, Hyland Division, Glendale, California, USA.

contracted for self-sufficiency with a commercial manufacturer). Many political agendas surround the issue of remunerated versus non-remunerated donors. The issue that appears most important is that of the quality and certification of the donor center(s). No difference in the safety, tolerability or efficacy of products derived from one or other type of donor center has been documented. Yield (the amount of IgG protein from 1 l of plasma) has been shown to vary by geographical distribution. Donor centers must maintain a high level of quality control in their testing laboratories, absolute matching of donor records with plasma donations (traceability), and provide virological follow-up analysis. Donors are given a medical examination, a complicated lifestyle analysis to screen out potential high-risk donations, and virological testing. Plasmapheresis donors are often repeat donors (> 75%) and usually donate more frequently than whole-blood donors. Some manufacturers prefer to use plasmapheresed donors in order to have greater standardization between lots of IVIg. All products today are produced from more than 1000 donors per lot, according to World Health Organization standards.

Appropriate screening of donors reduces the risks of viral transmission, but manufacturers must still employ methods of viral separation and inactivation to reduce these risks still further. The difficulty is that no single method of viral separation or inactivation is totally effective. Many manufacturers have only validated current purification methods, with respect to viral log reduction, without implementing more formal methods of destroying and/or eliminating potential viruses. Indeed, some manufacturers rely almost totally upon screening, e.g. polymerase chain reaction (PCR). Since 1 July 1999, hepatitis C antigen screening on the pooled plasma has been a requirement by the European authorities. The Americans have required hepatitis C antigen screening by PCR since 1995 for products that lack a formal virus inactivation step.

The basic problem with screening is that only known viruses may be screened for, and there is currently a lack of standardized testing methods and kits for most viruses. This lack of standardization results in different detection limits, false positives and false negatives. Besides the issue of detection limits, many assays are not validated by the assay manufacturers in the final IVIg products. The product itself or its excipients may cross-react, producing indeterminate or false results.

Three basic methods of primary viral inactivation are used by industry (Table 9.2). The use of solvent detergent is extremely effective against lipid-coated viruses, e.g. hepatitis C,[8–10] but has little activity against non-lipid coated viruses, e.g. parvovirus $B_{19}$. This method is gaining wide acceptance within the industry and with governmental regulatory authorities. Pasteurization is employed by only a few manufacturers. It is effective against those viruses sensitive to heat treatment at 60°C, but this excludes many viruses. Further, at 59°–61°C, the IgG molecule begins to denature, requiring extremely tight manufacturing controls. These manufacturers wrap the molecule in sugar to prevent damage. β-Propriolactone is used by one manufacturer. This method appears to be

**Table 9.2**
*Methods of viral inactivation and/or removal in the manufacture of intravenous immunoglobulin*

| Primary inactivation methods | Secondary inactivation methods | Separation methods |
| --- | --- | --- |
| Solvent detergent | pH 4 incubation | Cohn–Oncley fractionation |
| Pasteurization | Caprylic acid | Nanofiltration |
| β-Propriolactone | Addition of pepsin | Column chromatography |
| | Hydrolase treatment | Ion exchange |
| | Polyethylene glycol | Neutralizing antibodies |

the most effective against both lipid and non-lipid coated viruses, but unfortunately it significantly damages the Fc portion of the IgG molecule.

Because no single primary method is totally effective manufacturers employ additional secondary steps, including incubation at pH4, the addition of pepsin, caprylic acid, polyethylene glycol, and hydrolase treatment. Viral separation techniques are also employed by some firms, including nanofiltration, column chromatography, and the Cohn–Oncley fractionation steps. Still some viruses are extremely difficult to remove or kill, e.g. parvovirus $B_{19}$ and HAV. Therefore, some firms set minimum standards of antibody levels against these antigens to ensure neutralization. The FDA and the EC continue to examine this situation and propose new regulations.

In 1994 the German authorities proposed specific logarithmic reductions with multiple inactivation steps.[11] In 1995 these became only recommendations, after many members of industry and EC member states complained that compliance was not readily achievable. It is interesting to note that most companies are now able to comply with these stringent standards.

All three of the primary methods of inactivation are effective against hepatitis C and most lipid-coated viruses. The difficulty is with the inactivation and/or removal of non-lipid coated viruses, e.g. hepatitis A and parvovirus $B_{19}$. No effective process for the destruction of these viruses exists with today's commercial technology in IVIg.

Both parvovirus $B_{19}$ and HAV are susceptible to inactivation by exposure to high levels of heat treatment that would damage the IgG molecule, e.g. 100°C. Nanofiltration is only effective for the larger viruses, as the smallest effective filter that can be used is 35 nm (the diameter of the hepatitis A is approximately 27 nm, and that of parvovirus $B_{19}$ is 18–26 nm). Therefore, it is critical to ensure that the commercial IVIg preparations have adequate antibody levels of HAV and parvovirus $B_{19}$, to neutralize any antigen that may have contaminated the plasma pool. This neutralization process must be adequately validated by international standards.

Currently, validation of these methods is only partially standardized. Laboratories use model viruses because they are unable to grow enough of the actual virus, e.g. hepatitis C. There is no uniformity of model viruses by all manufacturers, and it is therefore very difficult to interpret some manufacturers' data. Clinicians should require manufacturers to show clear and understandable data with respect to viral safety, and should consult a virologist for interpretation of ambiguous information.

# Tolerability

The increased use of IVIg in the therapy of autoimmune disorders has accentuated the issue of tolerability. The literature containing adverse reactions to IVIg in clinical therapy ranges from 1% to 81%.[12,13] Although the majority of adverse reactions are mild and related to the speed of infusion, an increasing number of more serious reactions are emerging with the use of higher doses, for example cerebral infarction, acute renal failure, aseptic meningitis, myocardial infarction, thrombosis, arthritis, hyperviscosity and vasculitis.

The difficulty in determining the actual incidence is that most clinical studies are not designed to investigate tolerability, but rather to note adverse reactions. This has resulted in manufacturers reporting an incidence of 1–16% adverse reactions in their official prescribing information. This information on tolerability is rarely updated after the initial registration, unless mandated by a government authority. Authorities have recently begun to require pharmacovigilance studies. Clinicians should inquire as to the availability of such a report from the manufacturer. Before this time and at present, companies were required to file periodic safety reports and to immediately notify government officials of any serious reactions.

There does appear to be a significant difference between brands with respect to the global incidence of adverse reactions. This may be due to a large variance, with different pharmacological parameters between products. The majority of adverse reactions include headache, backache, nausea, vomiting, diarrhea, flushing, fever, chills, shaking, shortness of breath, tightness of the chest, hypotension, hypertension and rashes. These are usually transitory in nature and related to the speed of the infusion. Different products have slightly different rates of infusion because of their different stabilizers, total protein content and pH.

It is important that persons actually administering the IVIg read the manufacturer's package leaflet for the rate of infusion recommended for that specific product. Reactions usually occur within the first hour of the infusion. Should any of these reactions occur, stop the infusion, wait 30 minutes, and restart at a slower infusion speed. Even with the recommended infusion rate a large interpatient variability exists, such that some patients tolerate a much faster infusion speed and some require an even slower speed. Some patients may react even with very slow infusion speeds, and to different brands. These rare patients may require prophylaxis treatment 30 minutes before IVIg infusion with 50–100 mg hydrocortisone, an antipyretic, and/or an antihistamine.[14,15] With the exception of headache, which may occur up to 7 days post infusion, if these types of reactions occur at the end of the infusion or later, they may be related to pyrogen contamination of the product.

*In vivo* testing for pyrogens in rabbits, required by regulatory authorities for product release, is limited in dosing to the equivalent of 200–600 mg/kg. Dosing for autoimmune disorders is frequently higher or more prolonged than for immune replacement. Therefore, some manufacturers have instituted an *in vitro* limulus test to look more closely for pyrogen contamination. Only the *in vivo* testing is required by regulatory officials. Immediate reactions may also be due to the rapid formation of immune complexes in patients who have a concurrent infection, and it is generally advised that treatment be delayed until any infection has been treated or has resolved.

Additional reasons include the presence of aggregates, fragments, insoluble or incompletely dissolved lyophilate (in products requiring mixing before administration), the temperature of the solution being infused, and the total protein load being administered (some products contain albumin in addition to the IgG). Immunological reasons may include the triggering of an inflammatory response by product constituents; acute complement activation, with the production of anaphylatoxins C3a and C5a; triggering of mast cells and polymorphonuclear granulocytes, resulting in the release of histamine and other granule components; and

the release of tumor necrosis factor and other interleukins.[12,16–20]

Another type of early adverse reaction is specific to products with a pH below 5.0. These products may produce severe irritation and/or necrosis at the infusion site. The package leaflet of two different brands reports phlebitis and thrombotic complications. Neonates or those with impaired physiology may not be able to properly buffer the low pH if large doses are required. Severe headache has been documented in a number of neurological patients.[21,22]

Some headaches have been so severe as to require CT scans, which showed no evidence of intracranial hemorrhage.[23] Patients prone to headache or delayed-onset headache may require slowing of the infusion speed further, or the administration of low-dose β-blockers, which has sometimes been effective.[14] Aseptic meningitis has been reported in up to 11% of neurological patients receiving IVIg.[21] There is no evidence of subarachnoid hemorrhage, it is self-limiting and without major sequelae. Allogeneic IgG is known to cross the blood–brain barrier and elevated IgG levels of 1.5–7 times the upper limit of normal may be found in cerebrospinal fluid.[23] Aseptic meningitis may mimic bacterial meningitis, with neutrophilic pleocytosis, elevated protein concentration, and decreased glucose in the cerebrospinal fluid.[24] Treatment is symptomatic, with appropriate analgesics and antiemetics. However some centers begin antibiotic treatment because of the difficulty with a differential diagnosis, and base treatment time on IgG clearance from the cerebrospinal fluid. Patients with a history of migraine appear to be at a higher risk.[25] The mechanism is unknown, but may be due to a vasomotor effect on the meningeal microvasculature from an induced release of histamine, serotonin or prostagladins. Additional ideas are related to soluble molecules such as cytokines and human leukocyte antigens.

Arthritic complications have been described,[26] characterized by severe pain in multiple joints, especially the knees and wrists. Laboratory studies indicate elevated levels of circulating immune complexes as measured by binding to C3d, a mild decrease in serum C4 levels and a mild increase in total hemolytic complement. Potential mechanisms of action include the formation of specific antibody–antigen immune complex aggregates.

Acute renal failure is being seen more often with the high doses used in autoimmune patients. The products implicated contained high levels of sucrose as a stabilizer and have resulted in classic osmotic nephrosis.[22,27–29] Renal biopsy shows swelling and vacuolization of the proximal tubular epithelial cytoplasm, and IgG in the glomerulus. Creatinine may rise from 1.4 mg/dl to more than 6.5 mg/dl. Apart from the sucrose as a potential complicating factor, the osmolality may also

be contributing factor. Many manufacturers that produce lyophilized powders indicate that their products may be reconstituted at much higher concentrations than the standard 3% or 5%. At the standard concentrations, the osmolality is usually below 350 mmol. However, if a 6%, 10% or 12% concentration is made from these products, osmolality may rise to over 1000 mmol. This, in combination with higher sodium content in some products, may present problems in patients with underlying renal complications or diabetes, in neonates, and in patients over 60 years of age.

The osmolality issue may also be responsible for thrombogenesis secondary to hyperviscosity. Both cerebral infarction and myocardial infarction have been reported in older patients.[30–34] Plasma viscosity may rise by as much as 40%. Therefore, it is not recommended that products with an osmolality greater than 350 mmol be used in patients who may be sensitive to complications of hyperviscosity.

Additional complications have been associated with levels of isoagglutinins, anti-A, anti-B and anti-D. Products vary widely with regard to the content. Serum sickness without joint involvement and with immune hemolysis and disseminated intravascular coagulation has been reported as well as hemolytic anemia.[35–37] Clinicians should request the content of isoagglutinins for the products prescribed.

Rare dermatological events have been

reported.[22] These include eczema, erythema multiforme, purpuric erythema and alopecia. The mechanisms for these rare reactions are unknown.

Transient leukopenia[24] and neutropenia[38] have been reported. The leukopenia is normally asymptomatic. The neutropenia is rare. Proposed mechanisms of action include aggregates resulting in altered expression of cell surface CR3, thus causing adherence to blood vessels, the role of neutrophil FcR$\gamma$ III (CD64), and the presence in IVIg of antineutrophil antibodies.

Anaphylactic and anaphylactoid reactions are rare with IVIg, the majority of cases being reported in immunodeficient patients treated with IVIg. The reaction may be due to the formation of antibodies against IgA in patients with selective IgA deficiency (IgAD). The titer of anti-IgA antibodies does not correlate accurately with the risk of subsequent anaphylaxis; however, it is generally agreed that patients with high-titer anti-IgA antibodies should be carefully assessed before a supervised trial of a product low in IgA (products vary from 3 to 8000 µg/ml). If a reaction has been documented patients should be given advice regarding the risks with other blood products, and a Medic Alert bracelet documenting the risk. Table 9.3 lists the various adverse reactions known to be associated with IVIg.

**Table 9.3**
*Adverse reactions with intravenous immunoglobulins*

| *Mild* | *Moderate* | *Severe* |
|---|---|---|
| Headache | Headache | Aseptic meningitis |
| Bachache | Rashes | Acute renal failure |
| Nausea | Neutropenia | Cerebral infarction |
| Vomiting | Arthritis | Myocardial infarction |
| Diarrhea | Phlebitis | Hyperviscosity |
| Chills | Serum sickness | Thrombosis |
| Fever | Alopecia | Vasculitis |
| Shaking | Eczema | Hemolytic anemia |
| Flushing | Erythema multiforma | Disseminated intravascular coagulation |
| Hypertension | Leukopenia | Anaphylaxis reaction |
| Hypotension | Anaphylactoid reactions | |
| Tightness in the chest | Infusion site necrosis | |
| Shortness of breath | | |

## Conclusion

The majority of adverse reactions are mild and easily managed, but clinicians need to be aware of the potential complications of IVIg in regard to both viral safety and tolerability. Products vary significantly in their viral inactivation steps and pharmacological parameters. Clinicians should examine the choice of product(s) carefully with respect to these issues before assuming that all IVIg are generically the same. It appears that most IVIg are equally efficacious, but their safety and tolerability vary widely, which may result in severe morbidity and potential mortality.

## References


1.  Lane RS. Non-A non-B hepatitis from intravenous immunoglobulin. *Lancet* 1984; **ii:** 974–5.

2.  Lever AML, Webster ADB, Brown D, Thomas HC. Non-A, non-B hepatitis occurring in agammaglobulinaemic patients after intravenous immunoglobulin. *Lancet* 1984; **4:** 1062–4.

3.  Ochs HD, Fischer SH, Virant FS, et al. Non-A, non-B hepatitis after intravenous immunoglobulin. *Lancet* 1985; **i:** 404-5.

4.  Ochs HD, Fischer SH, Virant FS et al. Non-A, non-B hepatitis after intravenous immunoglobulin. *Lancet* 1986; **i:** 323. [Letter].

5.  Björkander J, Cunningham-Rundles C, Lundin P et al. Intravenous immunoglobulin prophylaxis causing liver damage in 16 of 77 patients with hypogammaglobulinemia or IgG subclass deficiency. *Am J Med* 1988; **84:** 107–11.

6.  Williams PE, Yap PL, Gillon J et al. Transmission of non-A, non-B hepatitis by pH 4.0 treated intravenous immunoglobulin. *Vox Sang* 1989; **57:** 15–18.

7.  Gomperts ED. Gammagard and reported hepatitis C virus episodes. *Clin Ther* 1996; **18**(Suppl. B): 3–8.

8.  Horowitz B, Prince AM, Hamman J, Watklevicz M. Viral safety of solvent/detergent-treated products. *Blood Coag Fibrinol* 1994; **5**(Suppl. 3): S21–8.

9.  Eriksson B, Westman L, Jernberg M. Virus validation of plasma-derived products produced by Pharmacia, with particular reference to immunoglobulins. *Blood Coag Fibrinol* 1994; **5**(Suppl. 3): S37–S44.

10.  Biesert L. Virus validation studies of immunoglobulin preparations. *Clin Exp Rheumatol* 1996; **14**(Suppl. 15): S47–S52.

11.  Paul-Ehrlich Institut, Bundesamt für Sera und Impfstoffe. Notice relating to measures against drug-associated risks. Reduction of the risk of transmission of hematogenous viruses in case of drugs manufactured by fractionation of plasma of human origin. *Bundesanzeiger* 1994.

12.  Weisman LE. The safety of intravenous immunoglobulin preparations. *Israel J Med Sci* 1994; **30:** 459–63.

13.  Bertorini TE, Nance AM, Horner LH, Greene W, Gelfand MS, Jaster JH. Complications of intravenous gammaglobulin in neuromuscular and other diseases. *Muscle Nerve* 1996; **19:** 388–91.

14.  Gelfand EW. Intravenous gammaglobulin therapy in immunocompromised patients. In: Garner RJ, Sacher RA, eds. *Intravenous Gammaglobulin Therapy*. Arlington, VA:

American Association of Blood Banks, 1988: 31–46.

15. Roberton DM, Hosking CS. Use of methylprednisolone as prophylaxis for immediate adverse infusion reactions in hypogammaglobulinaemic patients receiving intravenous immunoglobulin: a controlled trial. *Aust Paediatr J* 1988; **24:** 174–7.

16. Blasczyk R, Westhoff V, Grosse-Wilde H. Soluble CD4, CD8 and HLA molecules in commercial immunoglobulin preparations. *Lancet* 1993; **341:** 789–90.

17. Lam L, Whitsett CF, McNichol JM, Hodge TW. Immunologically active proteins in intravenous immunoglobulin. *Lancet* 1992; **342:** 678.

18. Mollnes TE, Høgåsen K, Hoaas BF, Michaelsen TE, Garred P, Harboe M. Inhibition of complement-mediated red cell lysis by immunoglobulins is dependent on the IG isotype and its C! binding properties. *Scand J Immunol* 1995; **41:** 449–56.

19. Mouthen L, Kaveri SV, Spalter SH et al. Mechanisms of action of intravenous immune globulin in immune-mediated diseases. *Clin Exp Immunol* 1996; **104**(Suppl. 1): 3–9.

20. Aukrust P, Müller F, Nordøy I, Haug CJ, Frøland SS. Modulation of lymphocyte and monocyte activity after intravenous immunoglobulin administration in vivo. *Clin Exp Immunol* 1997; **107:** 50–6.

21. Sekul EA, Cupler EJ, Dalakas MC. Aseptic meningitis associated with high-dose intravenous immunoglobulin therapy: frequency and risk factors. *Ann Intern Med* 1994; **121:** 259–62

22. Brannagan TH III, Nagle KJ, Lange DJ, Rowland LP. Complications of intravenous immune globulin in neurologic disease. *Neurology* 1996; **47:** 674–7.

23. Kattamis AC, Shankar S, Cohen A. Neurologic complications of treatment of childhood acute immune thrombocytopenic purpura with intravenously administered immunoglobulin G. *J Pediatr* 1997; **130:** 281–3.

24. Casteels-vanDaele M, Wijndaele L, Brock P, Kruger M, Gillis P. Aseptic meningitis associated with high-dose intravenous immunoglobulin therapy. *J Neurol Neurosurg Psychiatry* 1992; **55:** 980–1.

25. Vera-Ramirez M, Charlet M, Parry GJ. Recurrent aseptic meningitis complicating intravenous immunoglobulin therapy. *Neurology* 1992 **42:** 1636-7.

26. Lisak RP. Arthritis associated with circulating immune complexes following administration of intravenous immunoglobulin therapy in a patient with chronic inflammatory demyelinating polyneuropathy. *J Neurol Sci* 1996; **135:** 85–8.

27. Schifferli JA. High-dose intravenous immunoglobulin treatment and renal function. In: Dominioni L, Nydegger UE, eds. *Intravenous Immunoglobulins Today and Tomorrow.* London: Royal Society of Medicine Services Int. Congress and Symp Series, 1992; **189:** 27–33.

28. Ahsan N, Wiegand LA, Abendroth CS, Manning EC. Acute renal failure following immunoglobulin therapy. *Am J Nephrol* 1996; **16:** 532–6.

29. Hansen-Schmidt S, Silimon J, Keller F. Osmotic nephrosis due to high-dose immunoglobulin therapy containing sucrose (but not glycine) in a patient with immunoglobulin A nephritis. *Am J Kidney Dis* 1996; **28**(3): 451–3.

30. Ropper AH, Adelman L. Early Guillain–Barré syndrome without inflammation. *Arch Neurol* 1992; **49**: 979–81.

31. Silbert PL, Knezevic WV, Bridge DT. Cerebral infarction complicating intravenous immunoglobulin therapy for polyneuritis cranialis. *Neurology* 1992; **49**: 257–8.

32. Thornton CA, Ballow M. Safety of intravenous immunoglobulin. *Arch Neurol* 1993; **50**: 135–6.

33. Steg RE, Lefkowitz DM. Cerebral infarction following intravenous immunoglobulin therapy for myasthenia gravis. *Neurology* 1994; **44**: 1180.

34. Dalakas MC. High-dose intravenous immunoglobulin and serum viscosity: risk of precipitating thromboembolic events. *Neurology* 1994; **44**: 223–6.

35. Nakamura S, Yoshida T, Ohtake S, Matsuda T. Hemolysis due to high-dose intravenous gammaglobulin treatment for patients with idiopathic thrombocytopenic purpura. *Acta Haematol* 1986; **76**: 115–18.

36. Comenzo RL, Malachowski ME, Meissner HC, Fulton DR, Berkman EM. Immune hemolysis, disseminated intravascular coagulation, and serum sickness after large doses of immune globulin given intravenously for Kawasaki disease. *J Pediatr* 1992; **120**: 926–8.

37. Tamada KI, Kohga M, Masuda H, Hattori K. Hemolytic anemia following high-dose intravenous immunoglobulin administration. *Acta Paediatr Japon* 1995; **37**: 391–3.

38. Tam DA, Morton LD, Stroncek DF, Leshner RT. Neutropenia in a patient receiving intravenous immune globulin. *J Neuroimmunol* 1996; **64**: 175–8.

# Index

Note: Page numbers in **bold** refer to figures in the text; those in *italics* refer to tables or boxed material


acetylcysteine, 84

acute phase proteins, 67, 71

ADCC (antibody-dependent cell-mediated cytotoxicity), 5, 11, **13**

adhesion molecules, 12, 14, **15**, 27, 56, 59

adverse effects, 73–4, 94–5, 134, 137–41

    anaphylactic/anaphylactoid, 85, 94, 141

    arthritic, 140

    incidence, 47, 137–8

    and infusion rate, 122, 138, 139

    manufacturers' reporting, 138

    patient screening, 122

    urticaria, 47–8

    variation in products, 138, 139, 142

AECA (anti-endothelial cell antibodies), 69

allopurinol, 82

Alphaglobin, 49, 100, *102, 132*

anaemia, 67–8, 85

anaphylactic/anaphylactoid reactions, 85, 94, 141

ANCA (antineutropil cytoplasmic antibodies), 46, 69

aneurysms, arterial, 75

angio-oedema, 33

anti-BMZ antibody, **109**, 115

anti-factor VIIIc disease, 46

anti-FcER1 antibodies, 38, 44

anti-Forssman antibodies, 9–10

anti-idiotypic antibodies, 8–9, 46–7, 72

anti-IgA antibodies, 141

anti-IgE antibodies, 37–8, 39, 44

anti-TSH receptor antibodies, 101

antibody-dependent cell-mediated cytotoxicity (ADCC), 5, 11, **13**

anticonvulsant agents, 82

anti-endothelial cell antibodies (AECA), 69

antigens, opsonisation, 11, **12**

antihistamines, 40

antineutropil cytoplasmic antibodies (ANCA), 46, 69

α1-antitrypsin, 67, 71
apoptosis, 14–16, 59, 82–3, 85
arachidonic acid metabolism, 36
Arg-Gly-Asp antibodies, 14
Armoglobulina, *130*
arthritic complications, 140
aspirin, 36, 69, 71–2, *75*
atopic dermatitis
    incidence, 53
    IVIg mechanisms in, 58–9
    IVIg therapy, 6, 8, 54–8
autoantibodies
    bullous pemphigoid, **109**, 115
    cicatricial pemphigoid, 117
    downregulation, 6, 8
epidermolysis bullosa acquisita, 119–20
    Kawasaki disease, 69, 72
    neutralisation, 8–9
    pemphigus foliaceus, 113
    pemphigus vulgaris, 108, **109**
    pretibial myxoedema, 101
    urticaria, 37–8, 39, 46
autoantibody titres, 46, 123, 141
autoimmune mucocutaneous blistering
        diseases, 107–8
    indications for IVIg therapy, 123–4
    IVIg clinical data, *110*
    mechanisms of IVIg action, 122–3
    *see also individual diseases*

B cells
    antibody expression/secretion, 3, 5
    development, 2–3
    inhibition, 14, 72
bacterial superantigens, 12, 58–9, 68–9, 72
basement membrane zone autoantibodies,
        **109**, 115
basophils, 37–8, 39
β-propriolactone, 136
Biavin, *132*

blood screening, 122
blood-brain barrier, 97, 139
BP Ag1 autoantigen, 115
BP Ag2 autoantigen, 115, 121
bullous pemphigoid
    IVIg therapy, *110*, 115–17
    pathogenesis, **109**, 115

C3bNEO, 31
cardiological disease, 67, 73, 74–5
Careimune, *130*
CD5 antibodies, 6, 8
CD95 (Fas) antigen, 15, 83
cerebral infarction, 140
checklist, physician's, 95
chlormezanone, 82
chronic inflammatory demyelinating
        polyneuropathy (CIDP), 26, 96
cicatricial pemphigoid, *110*, 117–19
CIDP (chronic inflammatory demyelinating
        polyneuropathy), 26, 96
clofazamine, 98
colchicine, 99
collagen type VII autoantibodies, 119–20
complement system, 9
    dermatomyositis, 22–3, 30–1
    downregulation, 72–3
    neutralisation, 9–10
conjunctiva, 117–19
coronary artery disease, 67, 75
corticosteroids
    complications of use, 107–8, 115–16
    scleromyxoedema, 98
    synergism/sparing effects of IVIg, 16, 26,
        111, 114–15
    TEN and SJS, 84
    urticaria, 40
cyclophosphamide, 84, 120, 121
cyclosporin, 40, 84, 98, 120, 121
cytokines, 30, 72, 98–9, 123

atopic dermatitis, 55–6
Th1/Th2 balance, 12–14, 60
urticaria, 37
cytotoxic agents, 40, 84, 98, 120-1

dapsone, 120–1
dermatitis, atopic *see* atopic dermatitis
dermatomyositis
IVIg therapy
controlled study, 23–5, **30**
effects on muscle histology, 26–7, **28–9**
maintenance, 26
mechanisms of action, 26–7, 30–1
pathogenesis, 22–3
systemic sclerosis overlap, 99–100
desmoglein 1 autoantibodies, 108, 113
dipyridamole, 69, *75*
donors, 5, 135–6

E-selectin, 99
ECP *see* eosinophilic cationic protein
eczematous reactions, 47
ELAM-1 *see* endothelial leucocyte adhesion
molecule
encephalitis, in scleromyxoedema, 97
Endobulin Immuno, 101, *130*
endothelial leucocyte adhesion molecule 1
(ELAM-1), 56, 58, 59
eosinophilic cationic protein (ECP), 58, 60, 61
epidermolysis bullosa acquisita, *110*, 119–20
erythema multiforme, 80, *81*

Fab region, 11, *94*
Fas (CD95) antigen, 15, 83
Fas-FasL interaction, 59, 83, 85
Fc receptors, 5, *7*, 11, **12**, 46, 72, *94*
Flebogamma, *132*
Forssman antigen, 9–10

Gamimune, *131*

Gamma-Venin P, *130*
Gammagard, *130*, 135
Gammaraas, *133*
Gammar IVP, *130*
GammoNativ N, *131*
glucocorticoid receptor sensitivity, 16
glycosaminoglycans, dermal/subcutaneous
deposition, 100–1
Grave's disease, 100–1
growth factors, 99
Guillain-Barré syndrome, 31

$H_1$ receptor antagonists, 40
headache, 47, 85, 139–40
heart failure, congestive, 122
helper T (Th) cells, 12–14, 58
hepatitis C virus, 135, 136, 137
hepatitis A virus, 137
herpes gestationis, *110*, 121–2
herpes simplex virus, 82
HG factor, 121
histamine, 36
histamine-releasing autoantibodies, 37–8, 39,
46
HIV, 82, 122
HLA associations, 39, 82
Humaglobin, *133*
hydroxychloroquine, 55, 56
hypertension, 99, 122
hyperthyroidism, 100–1
hyperviscosity, 140
hypogammaglobinaemia, 98

IBM (inclusion body myositis), 21–2, 30
ICAM-1 (intercellular adhesion molecule-1),
27, 56, 58, 59
ICS (intercellular cement substance)
antibodies, 108, **109**
idiopathic thrombocytopenic purpura (ITP),
11, 46, 54–5, 69, 72, 85

IFN-γ (interferon-α), 13–14, 59
immunoglobulins, 2–5
    Fab fragments, 11, *94*
    isotypes, 3, *5*
    metabolic rate, 8
    structure, 3, **4**
immunosuppressive agents, 22, 108, 109
    *see also named agents*
*in vivo* testing, 138–9
inclusion body myositis (IBM), 21–2, 30
inflammatory myopathies, 21–2
infusion rate, 122, 138, 139
integrins, 14
intercellular adhesion molecule-1 (ICAM-1),
    27, 56, 58, 59
intercellular cement substance (ICS)
    antibodies, 108, **109**
interferon-α, 40
interferon-γ (IFN-γ), 13–14, 59
interleukin-1 (IL-1), 99, 123
interleukin-1 (IL-1) receptor antagonists, 123
interleukin-4 (IL-4), 13–14, 55–6
interleukin-5 (IL-5), 13–14
interleukin-6 (IL-6), 72
interleukin-10 (IL-10), 14
Intragam, *133*
Intraglobin CP, *131*
Intraglobin F, *131*
Isiven, *102, 132*
isoagglutins, 140
ITP (idiopathic thrombocytopenic purpura),
    11, 46, 54–5, 69, 72, 85

Kawasaki disease
    clinical features and diagnosis, 64–7, *68*,
        74
    epidemiology, 64
    first described, 63–4
    laboratory findings, 67–8
    long-term sequelae, 67, 73, 74–5
    mechanisms of IVIg action, 72–3
    pathogenesis, 68–9
    pathology, 68
    treatment
        adverse effects, 73–4
        current recommendations, 75–6
        IVIg, 54–5, 69, 71–2
        patients not fulfilling diagnostic criteria,
            74
        unresponsive patients, 73
keratinocyte apoptosis, 15–16, 59, 82–3, 85

LABD (linear IgA bullous disease), *110*,
    120–1
leucopenia, transient, 140–1
LFA-1 (lymphocyte function-associated
    antigen-1), 12
linear IgA bullous disease (LABD), *110*,
    120–1
liver enzymes, 47, 68
lymphocyte function-associated antigen-1
    (LFA-1), 12
lymphoproliferative disorders, 96
lyophilized powders, 140

macrophages, 11
    Fc receptors, 5, *7*, 11, **12**, 46, 72, *94*
malignancy, 87, 96
manufacture, 5–6
    viral inactivation, 136–7
mast cell mediators, 36–7, 39
mast cells, 36, 39
mechanisms of action, 6–16, 94, 122–3, 134
    anti-idiotypic antibodies, 8–9, 46–7, 72
    B cells, *7*, 14, 72
    cell adhesion, *7*, 14, **15**, 27, 56, 59
    complement system, 9–10, 22–3, 30–1,
        72–3
    cytokines, 12–14, 30, 55–6, 72, 98–9, 123
    Fc receptor, 5, *7*, 11, 46, 72, *94*

glucocorticoid receptor, 16, 26, 111,
    114–15
  superantigens, 58–9
  T cells, 11–12, 14–15, 56, 58, 82–3
membrane attack complex (MAC), 9–10,
    22–3, 30–1
memory cells, 3
meningitis, aseptic, 47, 85, 94, 139
MHC class I molecule, 23, 27, **29**
MHC class II molecule, 68–9, **70**
minocycline, 98
mucous membrane (cicatricial) pemphigoid,
    *110*, 117–19
myasthenia gravis, 31
*Mycoplasma pneumoniae*, 82
myocardial infarction, 140
myocardial ischaemia, 67, 75
myopathies, inflammatory, 21–2
    *see also* dermatomyositis
myxoedema, pretibial, 100–3

neonatal herpes gestationis, 121
neutropenia, transient, 140–1
Nikolsky sign, 80
nodular pemphigoid, 115
non-steroidal anti-inflammatory agents, 82
Nottingham Health Profile, 34–5

Octagam, *102, 131*
ocular pemphigus, 117–19
oesophageal sclerosis, 100
opsonisation, 11, **12**
oral pemphigoid, **118**, 119
osmolality, 140
osmotic nephrosis, 140

Panglobulin, *130*
pansclerotic morphoea of childhood, 100
paraproteins, 96
parvovirus B$_{19}$, 137

pasteurization, 136
patient
  blood screening, 122
  checklist, 95
pemphigus foliaceus, *110*, 113–15
pemphigus vulgaris, 108–13
  adjunctive therapy, 111
  incidence, 108
  IVIg therapy, 109–13
  pathogenesis, 108
D-penicillamine, 99
pentoxyphylline, 84, 98
pH, 139
pharmacology, 129–34
phenobarbitol, 85
plasma viscosity, 140
plasmapheresis, 22, 46, 84, 115, 121
platelet count, 67, 71, 72
Polyglobin, *102, 131*
Polyglobulin, *130*
polymyositis, 22
polyneuropathy, chronic inflammatory
    demyelinating (CIDP), 26, 96
pompholyx eczema, 47
prednisolone, 55, 56, 98, 100
pregnancy, 121–2
pretibial myxoedema, 100–3
products (IVIg)
  osmolality, 140
  pH, 139
  pharmacological data, *130–3*
  variation in adverse effects, 138, 139, 142
  variation in efficacy, 45–6, 134
pyoderma gangrenosum, 97–9, 101–3
pyrogen contamination, 138–9
quality of life, 124

rash, 47
Raynaud's phenomenon, 100
renal dysfunction, 85, 88

renal failure, 99, 140

Sandoglobulin, 47, 98, *102, 130*
sclerodactyly, 100
scleroderma *see* systemic sclerosis (SSc)
scleromyxoedema, 95–7, 101–3
SCORTEN, 88
screening
    donors, 135–6
    patients, 122
self Sufficiency, *133*
serum sickness, 140
skin pigmentation changes, 100
solvent detergent, 136
SSC, (systemic sclerosis) 99–100, 101–3
Stevens-Johnson syndrome (SJS), 79
    causative drugs, 80, 82, 83
    clinical features, 80, *81*
    management, 83–8
    mortality, 82
    overlap with TEN, *81*
sulphapyridine, 120–1
sulphonamides, 82
superantigens, 12, 58–9, 68–9, 72
synergistic effects, 16, 26
systemic sclerosis (SSc), 99–100, 101–3

T cells, 2, 59, 72
    CD4$^+$, 11, 12–14, 56, 58, 82
    CD8$^+$, 12–13, 56, 82
    inhibition by IVIg, 11–12
    modulation of proliferation, 14–15
    superantigen activation, 68–9, **70**, 72
    toxic epidermal necrolysis, 82–3
T-cell receptor, 69, **70**
Tegeline, *132*
TEN *see* toxic epidermal necrolysis
TGF-β (transforming growth factor-α), 30,
    99

thalidomide, 84
thrombogenesis, 140
tissue fibrosis, 99
TNF-α (tumour necrosis factor-α), 72
toxic epidermal necrolysis (TEN), 79
    causative drugs, 80, 82, 83
    clinical features, 80, **81**
    incidence, 80, 82
    management
        IVIg therapy, 84–9
        prevention of disease progression, 83–4
        supportive treatment, 83
    mortality, 82
    pathogenesis, 82–3
    SJS overlap, *81*
transforming growth factor-β (TGF-β), 30,
    99
tumour necrosis factor-α (TNF- α), 72

urticaria, 33
urticaria, chronic
    clinical features, 34–5
    current treatments, 40
    evidence for autoimmune aetiology, 39
    'idiopathic', 34
    IVIg adverse effects, 47–8
    IVIg therapy, 40–5
    pathogenesis, 35–40
    pathogenetic subsets, 39–40

Venimmun, *130*
Venoglobulin S, 101, *102, 132*
vesicular hand eczema, 47
Viagam Liquid, *132*
Viagam-S, *131*
viral inactivation, 136–7
viral transmission, 122, 134–7

white cell count, 67